The Demise of Our Healthcare
We can prevent it

Rachot Vacharathone, MD

AHM Publishing, LLC
Salt Lake City

AHM Publishing, LLC
AHM Copyright, LLC
PO Box 1000
Draper, UT 84020

www.healthcaredemise.com

Design and composition by Ryan Christensen, American Printing and Promotion
Cover design by Ryan Christensen, American Printing and Promotion

Vacharothone, MD, Rachot
 The demise of our healthcare: we can prevent it

p. cm.

Includes bibliographical references.
ISBN-13: 978-0-615-85581-3

Printed in the United States of America

First Printing, November 7, 2013

*This book is dedicated to
all of my staff at After Hours Medical clinics
who are devoted to
their patients and their communities.*

Contents

Acknowledgments

Acknowledgements

There are many people who have come into my life and have shined a bright light into who I am and what my purpose is for humanity. I am thankful to have come into contact with many of you, my colleagues, my friends, and my family.

I want to especially thank the two most important people in my life, my mother and my father. They sacrificed the ability to be close to their son at the age of 13 for the desire for me to be the best that I could be. They taught me what I needed to know during my first 13 years, so I could be on my own in a far away land thereafter. If it were not for them asking me the magic question, "Son, do you want to go to the United States and become a doctor?" I would not be where I am today. I am deeply appreciative of the sacrifice they have made. This book, therefore, is written for them.

Two more very important people in my life are my aunt Kay and my uncle Doctor Somsak who, without hesitation, took me into their lives and provided me with the start that I needed to succeed in my education in the United States. Were it not for them, I would not be here helping my patients, writing this book, and sharing with the rest of the nation my ideas on how we can save our healthcare system together.

Last but not least are my wife and two children who have always been there to support me throughout my venture into the challenging world of healthcare. They have been so patient. They give me the daily energy I need to make things happen.

Introduction

We Can Prevent It

Our private healthcare system is broken.

Increasing medical care costs and higher insurance premiums will push more and more people with private insurance to financial ruin.

The combination of paying for high insurance premiums and paying additional out-of-pocket costs is imposing more financial strain on individuals, families, employees, and employers to the point where many just cannot make it financially. At some point in the near future, health insurance premiums will become so high that there will not be enough funds to pay for the healthcare expenses for everyone as Obamacare (the Patient Protection and Affordable Care Act) has planned. This is because paying the penalty for not complying with the new healthcare law is cheaper than buying health insurance.

Obamacare has several important features that our broken healthcare needs. Nonetheless, working alone, the Obamacare law and its mandate will only make this problem worse as long as it continues to lack effective control of medical care costs, despite the limitation already placed on the profit margins of health insurance companies. Meanwhile, Americans are becoming less healthy as these costs increase, while lack of competition in the health insurance market prevents creation of enough new competitive health plans that can help reduce consumers' costs.

As long as there is no effective medical care cost control and a lack of sufficient competition in the insurance market, the end results are: a sicker population, increasing deaths, more financially strained families and small businesses, and increasing medical bankruptcy—all constituting what I call The Demise of Our Healthcare, thus the title of this book.

However, *we*—you and I, the healthcare providers and the healthcare consumers of this country—can do something to prevent this death before it becomes too late. Otherwise, total governmental control of our healthcare system will be unavoidable.

Have you ever stopped and wondered why you pay so much for health insurance, have never had to use it for a major medical emergency, and yet keep on paying for it at an ever increasing price? Have you ever added up the monthly premiums that you have paid over the years and figured out how much you would have earned had a part of that fund been put away in investment accounts with compound interest? Have you ever considered what kind of improvements you could have made to your standard of living, such as home life and leisure activities, had your health insurance not cost so much?

These days people are not only wondering why their premiums are so high but also why they increase every year. Many of these people rarely use the healthcare system at all.

Despite the annual increases in health insurance premiums, we have to pay more when seeing a doctor. Haven't we paid enough in premiums already so we can avoid such out-of-pocket costs? Isn't this the very purpose of having health insurance? Why should we still continue to pay more each year? And what will the future look like?

Then there are those 49 million or so people living in this country who are uninsured. Is it because they cannot afford it? The answer is probably not for all. Many of them elect to be uninsured so they can hold on to thousands of dollars over the years for more tangible necessities rather than for the peace of mind of having health insurance. Welcome to our American Healthcare system.

After having paid so much for our insurance plans so we can receive the care we need and avoid financial setback in medical emergencies, some of us still end up with either one of the two worst possible outcomes—medical bankruptcy or death.

Yes, our private healthcare system is clearly broken. Our medical care costs have skyrocketed. For many decades we have received medical services without knowing their prices, and now we buy increasingly expensive health insurance to help with these increasing costs, only to encounter the two worst outcomes we hoped to prevent in the first place, thus defeating the purpose of having health insurance.

Now things are clearly changing for the worse. Again, working alone, Obamacare will allow the medical care costs and insurance premiums to skyrocket, leading to more undesirable outcomes.

But there is hope.

There are three problems that contribute to increasing healthcare costs and deceasing returns. Once these problems are understood, you will see that there are actions we can take to help turn our healthcare system around. We, the people, can regain control of our healthcare system and then receive medical care at affordable prices again.

That is what this book is all about. This book discusses our private healthcare system (not governmental plans such as Medicaid, Medicare, and their associated problems) simply because it is the only system in which we can come together, take action, and make changes for the better.

This book is for healthcare consumers and healthcare providers. It explains the suffering and the negative effects the recent changes in our healthcare system are having on all of us, particularly patients and our good old family doctors. It describes the three main interrelated problems that contribute to the crisis. Then it explains the cause of these three problems.

In the end, this book explains how we can take control and work together, in conjunction with the Obamacare and insurance companies, to improve our private healthcare system and to prevent further unwanted outcomes and, for that matter, its demise. We must take action before our government tries to help out even more, Obamacare being a prime example.

However, one may ask, what is wrong with a government-backed healthcare system? It works for other countries such as Sweden, Switzerland,

and Canada where everyone is entitled to free medical care. And after all, we do have a good example of the most government-controlled healthcare system right here in our own backyard, the Veteran's Administration (VA) healthcare system. Why can't we turn the rest of our system into one like the VA where everyone is entitled to medical care for little or no cost?

The answer is simple—we can if we simply give up. But if we give up, we will risk losing the ability to choose healthcare services freely. After all, one only has to enter a VA hospital to discover how limiting medical options can be. If we sit back and let the current tide of healthcare sweep us away, then the rest of our healthcare system may become like the VA. Do we really want such a system in our free enterprise economy and in this country where freedom of choice is our most valued privilege? If not, we *must* do something to prevent it.

As the contents in this book become understood and accepted throughout our country, we all can take steps in conjunction with Obamacare to create a healthcare revolution. We can reset the purpose of our healthcare system to what it used to be and allow the system to start providing high-quality, affordable medical services once again. In the meantime, we maintain the freedom to choose as patients and the freedom to provide as doctors.

One

CHAPTER 1
In a Nutshell

What's Wrong with this Picture?

Going through our daily lives during this time of economic hardship is like walking on a narrow rope bridge with wooden steps set far apart. To get to the other side, one must be careful with every step, making sure not to misstep or make any unexpected moves that could result in losing one's balance and a subsequent fall.

This is why we buy insurance for our family and ourselves. In case we encounter unexpected medical emergencies, we have a safety net that catches us and allows us to continue our lives without undue financial duress. Good insurance is like a net that is set close to each of these wooden steps so any misstep can result in a quick recovery.

However, have you noticed that despite having "good" health insurance, unexpected health events these days can still result in financial disaster, or at least a greater financial hardship from which it is difficult to recover?

In my 15-year career as an urgent care physician, supervising more than three hundred medical doctors, physician's assistants, nurse practitioners, and nursing staff, I have encountered countless patient cases that led me to look further into our broken healthcare system. I wanted to try to make sense of the problems, what the causes might be, and what we can do now to fix them. I wanted to know what the public could do to help, as opposed to waiting for insurance entities or our government to finally come to the rescue. This is the reason I wrote this book.

A couple of situations illustrate how my interest was piqued.

Kidney Stone

Karen H. (pseudonym) is my personal banker at a local bank. One day she approached me as I walked into the branch and asked, "Do you want to know what happened to me last month?"

Not having a primary care doctor she could conveniently access, Karen checked into a local emergency room because of pain on the right side of her back. She had had similar pain in the past and it had been due to a kidney stone. This time she thought it was another kidney stone, and so did the ER nurse who took care of her. The nurse said, "This pain is classic for a kidney stone!"

It turned out that Karen received the best of medical care that an emergency room can offer for a potential kidney stone. The ER doctor immediately ordered four blood tests, a urinalysis, IV fluid therapy, and a CT scan of the abdomen looking for kidney stones. When the CT scan did not reveal any kidney stones, an ultrasound was ordered which was also negative. She was then given medication for pain control, with a diagnosis of presumed kidney stone. She apparently passed a small stone the following day and her back pain resolved.

What came several days later in the mail was a statement from the hospital, detailing all the charges billed to her insurance company as demonstrated in Table 1.

So, Karen went into this emergency room and received a $7,520 state-of-the-art work up for a simple kidney stone attack, which is a typical approach for taking care of a kidney stone patient in an ER. Such a visit would have cost much less at a regular doctor's office with a less aggressive approach. She ended up paying $125 out of pocket for this ER trip instead of paying just a copay of $20 to $40 at a doctor's office for a simple kidney stone evaluation, in addition to more than $7,000 billed to her insurance instead of less than $200.

Procedures	Charge Amount ($)
Emergency room facility fee	1,711.00
CT scan	3,365.00
Ultrasound	1,072.00
Lab tests:	
Blood draw fee	122.00
Chemistry	442.00
Immunology	101.00
Hematology	79.00
Microbiology	190.00
Urology	120.00
IV therapy	191.00
Pharmacy	64.00
Supplies	63.00
Total Charges	$7,520.00

Table 1. Charges for procedures performed for presumed kidney stone in Karen's case.

Let me explain. Evaluating and treating a kidney stone patient at a doctor's office costs much less than at an ER because of the conservative approach taken. A kidney stone attack usually has a typical presentation and can be "clinically" diagnosed through two clinical findings: tenderness of the back over the kidney on examination, and the finding of red blood cells in the urine by a simple urinalysis test. This is usually the approach taken at a doctor's office.

While ordering a CT scan in a patient with kidney stone is a common approach in an ER, a CT scan or an ultrasound is not indicated to make the diagnosis at a regular doctor office during the initial visit. This is because most kidney stones are too small to be detected by a CT scan and will pass on their own. So the initial approach at a doctor's office for a kidney stone patient is to make a presumed, clinical diagnosis and then treat it with pain control and increasing fluid intake to help make the stone pass quickly for the next 48 hours. This constitutes a conservative but reasonable standard of care, one which would have cost a $20 to $40 copay at a regular doctor office, and $7,000 less than the ER charge.

A CT scan or an ultrasound is not needed until later if the stone does not pass within 48 hours and the pain does not subside. At that later time, it would then be appropriate to perform a CT scan to see how big the stone is. This would determine whether or not a referral to a urologist would be warranted in order to retrieve the stone with an instrument or break it up with lithotripsy, an ultrasonic method of disintegrating kidney stones.

From a cost perspective, the conservative standard used at a doctor's office or an urgent care clinic would have been the preferred approach for Karen's medical care. But due to convenience and today's trend toward use of state-of-the-art facilities for diagnosis and treatment, she received care from an ER that was unnecessarily costly.

One may argue that such an aggressive approach may be necessary in certain cases of unbearable pain or life-threatening presentation of kidney stone attack. However, despite the severe pain that a kidney stone can present, the pain is always controllable to a certain degree and it is not life threatening unless there is an associated infection or a blockage of the passage of urine, in which case the symptoms will worsen in the next 24 to 48 hours, at which time the patient would be referred to a specialist. This is the same two-day-later process both the ER and a primary care doctor would follow anyway.

This actual patient case demonstrates the lack of convenient primary care access and the use of aggressive medicine, two of the major problems in our healthcare system today.

Bell's Palsy

Nuntida B. (pseudonym) is my aunt who lives in Florida. One day the entire right side of her face became numb and droopy. She was not able to close her right eye. She went to a doctor who thought that she might have a condition called Bell's Palsy—a temporary paralysis of a facial nerve that is self-resolving and leaves no residual complications. However, the doctor also said, "There is a small chance that this could be a stroke. So let's do a CT scan of your brain."

The doctor ordered an outpatient CT scan of the brain in a nearby clinic, which showed a small circular spot that appeared abnormal to the doctor. He then told my aunt, "There may be bleeding in the brain." So Nuntida was sent to the hospital that shared a campus with the clinic and the outpatient CT scan clinic—one might wonder if the clinic, the outpatient CT clinic, and the hospital were owned by the same company or not, and who stood to profit from the many procedures subsequently ordered for Nuntida.

After arriving at the emergency room, she was seen by an ER physician who spent about ten minutes examining her and immediately initiated a

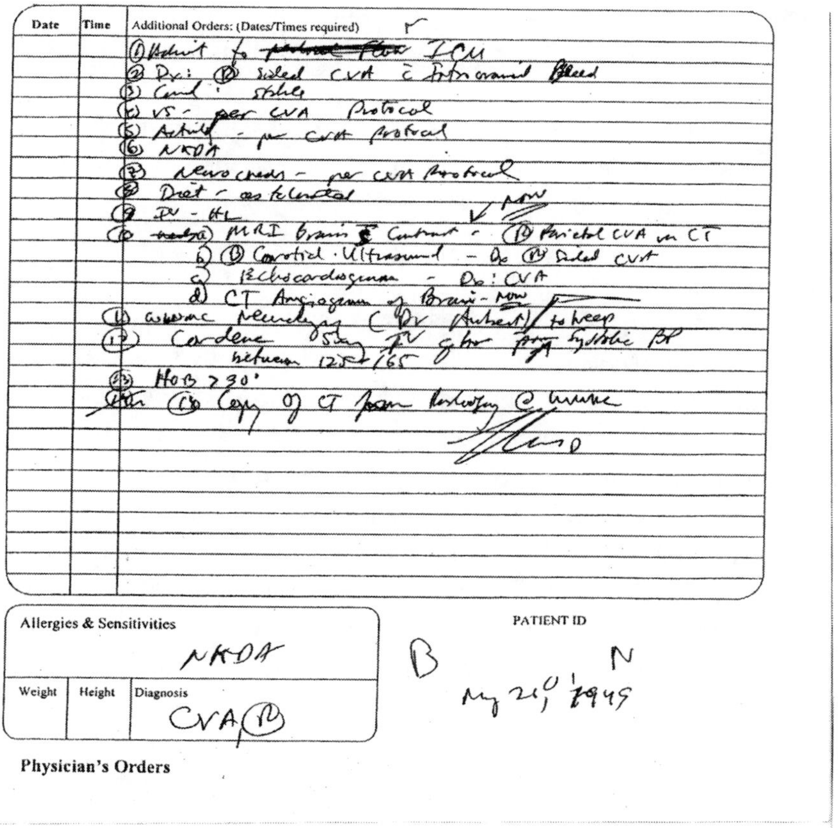

Date	Time	Additional Orders: (Dates/Times required)
		1) Admit to ICU
		2) Dx: (R) Sided CVA c̄ Intracranial Bleed
		3) Cond: stable
		4) VS - per CVA Protocol
		5) Activity - per CVA Protocol
		6) NKDA
		7) Neuro checks - per CVA Protocol
		8) Diet - as tolerated
		9) IV - HL
		10) a) MRI Brain c̄ Contrast - (R) Parietal CVA on CT — now
		b) (B) Carotid Ultrasound - Dx (R) Sided CVA
		c) Echocardiogram - Dx: CVA
		d) CT Angiogram of Brain - now
		11) Consult Neurology (Dr [illegible]) to keep
		12) Cardene 5mg IV q1hr prn Systolic BP between 125-165
		13) HOB > 30°
		14) Copy of CT from Radiology @ clinic

Allergies & Sensitivities: NKDA

Weight	Height	Diagnosis
		CVA, (R)

PATIENT ID

Physician's Orders

Illustration 1. This is the actual medical record showing the doctor's order in admitting my aunt to the ER for further care.

stroke treatment protocol by writing out a list of orders in his medical notes, as shown in Illustration 1.

After these orders were entered, nothing happened. Nuntida waited in an exam room and wondered who was going to come and see her next. After an hour she decided to call her daughter to help out. Her daughter then called the ER and asked why her mom was left waiting, having potentially suffered a stroke, and why no one had attended to her for more than an hour. Finally a nurse started an IV and carried out the doctor's order to draw blood, before proceeding with two additional brain scans. A portable chest x-ray was also performed.

Instead of consulting the outpatient CT scan already performed, the ER physician put my aunt through *another* CT scan, this one located inside the hospital. Additionally, instead of waiting for the result of that second CT scan, my aunt was wheeled straight into an MRI scanning room for another brain scan.

My poor aunt was stressed and anxious, thinking she was having a stroke that could leave her with permanent disabilities. Little did she know (because no one bothered to tell her) that her brain MRI was normal, as was the second brain CT scan performed before the MRI.

After the MRI Nuntida was left waiting in a hallway for another two hours. To her surprise, after fearing that she was dying from a stroke, someone other than her ER physician found her waiting in the hallway and asked why she was still in the hospital. This person told her the MRI was negative for a stroke and that she could go home.

My aunt was finally discharged with a diagnosis of Bell's Palsy. She never saw the ER physician again. Clearly this doctor should have come back and explained the Bell's Palsy diagnosis to her and given her instructions. Upon discharge, a nurse handed her prescriptions for a steroid and an antiviral medication, a typical treatment for Bell's Palsy. Two weeks later her facial paralysis and inability to close her right eye resolved and she went back to her normal life.

In analyzing this case, what is the most bothersome is that not only were two additional scans ordered (CT and MRI), but the ER physician also ordered a shotgun "cocktail" of blood tests and treatments for both diagnoses of hemorrhagic stroke (bleeding in the brain) and Bell's Palsy—one being life threatening, while the other completely self-resolving. These orders included:

- Starting IV fluid.
- Giving Nitroprusside, an IV medication to lower her blood pressure.
- Drawing her blood for complete blood count (CBC, showing red blood cells, white blood cells, and platelets), chemistry (showing blood levels of sodium, potassium, and other chemicals), and PT & PTT (showing blood clotting factors and clotting time).
- Giving IV steroid (to treat the Bell's Palsy).
- Giving Valtrex, an anti-viral medication for the Bell's Palsy.

In his charting, as shown in Illustration 2, the ER doctor wrote "hemorrhagic stroke" (bleeding in the brain) as the diagnosis and additionally ordered admission to ICU, a CT scan, an MRI scan, *as well as* an ultrasound of the carotid arteries and an echocardiogram of the heart. What is wrong here is that the carotid artery ultrasound and the echocardiogram of the heart could not have been the correct procedures to order because these are used to look for clots in the arteries and the heart that could have been dislodged to the brain, causing a "clotting stroke." My aunt's diagnosis, according to the doctor, was "bleeding stroke," not stroke from blood clots, therefore incorrect procedures were ordered. Luckily the carotid ultrasound and the echocardiogram were never performed. The ER physician also ordered a consultation from a neurologist whom my aunt claimed she never saw. And although documentation of the neurologist's visit never existed, a charge and payment for his consultation appeared on her bill, as shown on Table 2.

Here are some questions about my aunt's medical care that makes one think profit-making could have been the goal of treatment:

- Why perform two CT scans?
- Why go straight to an MRI after two CT scans without reviewing the existing CT scans and evaluating its necessity?
- Why perform a portable chest x-ray on a stroke patient? (This is unwarranted because stroke patients do not have any related or causative processes going on in the lungs.)
- Why obtain a neurology consult when all of the tests had been ordered and the treatment would remain the same?
- Why treat both the stroke and the Bell's Palsy at the same time?

Description	Charges ($)	Insurance Paid ($)	Patient Balance ($)
Clinic visit (family doctor)	103.00	88.30	0.00
Out-patient CT scan	367.00	0.00	301.44
ER facility fee	1,250.00	1,000.00	250.00
ER doctor fee	210.00	210.00	0.00
Neurology consult in ER	347.00	0.00	284.97
Subtotal	2,277.00	1,298.30	836.41
Hospital charges:			
IV medications	2,425.00	1,940.00	430.72
PO medications (by mouth)	134.00	107.20	0.00
Chemistry blood test	842.00	673.60	0.00
Clotting blood test PTT	409.00	327.20	0.00
Clotting blood test PT	317.00	253.60	0.00
Complete blood count (CBC)	440.00	352.00	0.00
Blood draw fee	57.00	45.60	0.00
Chest X-ray, portable 1 view	529.00	423.20	0.00
X-ray reading fee	34.00	0.00	12.80
CT scan of brain	3,927.00	3,141.60	0.00
CT reading fee	218.00	0.00	81.32
MRI scan of brain	4,052.00	3,241.60	0.00
MRI reading fee	285.00	0.00	106.43
Subtotal	13,669.00	10,505.60	631.27
Total	$15,946.00	$11,803.90	$1,467.68

Table 2. Summary of charges and payments for procedures performed on my aunt for a Bell's Palsy visit.

The sad point about my aunt's experience, which illustrates similar experiences of many other Americans, is that she could have received medical care from a good old family doctor for her Bell's Palsy for a small fee. Look at the cost of her doctor visit at the top of the summary:

Description	Charges	Insurance Paid	Patient Paid
Clinic visit	$103	$88.30	0

The costs could have and should have stopped there. In other words the costs incurred in my aunt's case are spurious for several reasons. The "spot on her brain" that incurred significant cost for her treatment was due to a calcification that is commonly seen in older patients. Such calcification usually has a characteristic circular appearance on a CT scan and should not be mistaken for bleeding. Had the first CT scan been read properly, before moving forward with another CT scan and the MRI and all of the other unnecessary treatments, the treatment would have stopped at merely

prescribing three inexpensive medications and issuing some simple
instructions:

- A steroid for reducing inflammation of the trigeminal nerve ($4 at
  a local pharmacy for the entire prescription).
- An antiviral medication because Bell's Palsy is associated with
  viral infection of the trigeminal nerve (also $4 at a local pharmacy).
- Artificial tears because the eyelid is paralyzed temporarily.
- Instruction to rest at home with taping of the paralyzed eyelid at
  night to prevent the eye from drying.

Had the three doctors (especially the mysterious neurologist) recognized
the classic presentation of Bell's Palsy, which has been easily and commonly
recognized since 1829, then $15,946 in unnecessary total charges could have
been avoided and my aunt would have saved $1,467.68 plus a day of anxious
waiting in the hospital.

Both Karen and my aunt received too little basic care and far too much
unnecessary and expensive advanced care. Countless other cases such as
these have made US healthcare the most expensive in the world without
better outcomes.

Death Without Insurance and Even with Insurance

We live in a nation that has the most advanced medical technology in the
world. Because of such privilege, we hope that our people do not die from
basic medical problems such as strep throat or from a complex illness like
liver failure. However, some do die for trivial reasons.

In the past, my clinics used to see patients coming in soon after the onset
of a head cold and sore throat. These days, we are seeing patients presenting
with full-blown pneumonia, advanced sinus infections, or severe infections
of the ears, throat, lungs, or kidneys because they do not come in earlier
for detection and treatment. They wait until their head cold turns into a
sinus infection, or the infection has already traveled into their lungs. We see
patients' health deteriorate due to a failure to visit their primary care doctors
regularly and from not taking their prescriptions. They end up in our urgent

care clinics with full-blown complicated medical problems. These patients are delaying care because their health plans offer less coverage, higher copays, higher deductibles, or because they have no health insurance at all.

One particular case was a patient named John H. (pseudonym), a previously healthy 35-year-old man, who had no health insurance. He presented to one of my clinics for an illness that started four weeks prior to the visit. He started having symptoms of a head cold that turned into green drainage from his sinuses. Three weeks after the onset, he started having a sore throat and decreased energy. Then he came into the clinic. The rapid strep test was negative at the clinic; in such an event, it is common to send out for a more elaborate strep culture. The patient did not want a strep culture sent out because of the cost and because he did not have health insurance. Our doctor prescribed him an antibiotic for a presumed bacterial infection anyway because of the length of the illness and the worsening of his symptoms. The doctor stressed the importance of taking the medication.

One week later the patient died. The death certificate reported "probable Streptococcal sepsis" as the cause of death. A family member reported that the patient never filled his prescription due to the cost. The family had also encouraged the patient to seek help earlier but he refused due to having no health insurance. I was very saddened by the case.

According to a Harvard Medical School study published by American Journal of Public Health on September 17, 2009, lack of health insurance was responsible for about 45,000 preventable deaths in the US in 2009. Since then, as the number of uninsured rose from about 46.3 million in 2009 to 48.6 million in 2011, the number of preventable deaths due to lack of insurance had grown to about 48,000 per year, according to Physicians for a National Health Program published on September 12, 2012.

On the other end of the spectrum, patients with life-threatening illnesses who have health insurance can still die due to denial of coverage for lifesaving procedures by their insurance carriers. A perfect example of such denied care resulting in death is 17-year-old Natalie Sarkisyan described in Wendall Potter's book *Deadly Spin*. She suffered from end-stage liver failure. She was waiting for a liver transplant to save her life but ended up dying a few hours after her health insurance finally gave in and approved a transplant procedure. Her health insurance had denied the coverage for the transplant for several days only to relent under negative media publicity in the end—when it was too late to save her life.

"Houston, We Have a Problem Problems!"

The case studies discussed above demonstrate the three fundamental problems of our current healthcare system in the private sector:

- The underuse of basic medicine
- The overuse of money-making medicine
- Profit-driven health insurance

The magnitude of such problems, extending nationwide, is unimaginable. These are only four examples in hundreds of thousands of similar cases. These three fundamental problems are amplified when viewing healthcare as a whole. They lead down an inevitable path of skyrocketing medical care costs and higher insurance premiums without an end in sight.

Ultimately the only solution for controlling premiums and medical care costs may be for our government to step in and be more involved in our private healthcare system altogether, as Obamacare is already attempting to do. At that time, private health insurers may leave the market because of even stricter regulations and less profits, as well as individuals and companies not buying insurance and paying penalties instead. Then our hospitals and medical doctors will have to deal directly with total government-controlled insurance providers. But is this the ideal solution? Of course not. This book will explore alternate solutions that you and I can create together—solutions that will help Americans retain their private healthcare system in which health insurance companies do not have to leave the market and our hospitals continue to deal with private health plans instead of governmental health plans exclusively.

Underuse of Basic Medicine

The biggest problem that we have in our country is that we don't know our doctors anymore. What happened to the good old family doctors that many of us used to know by first name? Now many of us don't see the same doctors over the course of our lifetimes. We either "don't have time" for them or our insurance has changed so many times that we are forced to see multiple doctors. Consequently many Americans have opted to care for their own health by taking over-the-counter medications, delaying care for perceived "minor illnesses," or simply walking into ERs.

What happens when we don't go to the doctor for regular checkups? What happens when we don't get into a clinic to take care of our sinus infection that could turn into pneumonia later if not treated now? We become unhealthy. We get sick easier. Then what do we do? We open our insurance booklets to find a doctor's number, make a call, and wait a few days for an appointment. We also notice that there are many specialists and facilities we can go to, some being more convenient to visit than waiting for an appointment with a primary care doctor. Why? The number of primary care doctors is declining. There are fewer doctors upon whom we can call for advice, doctors who know us by name and who are familiar with our medical history without having to open up our charts.

Ultimately we end up walking into an ER or a specialist's clinic for our medical needs. We will inevitably pay more than when such help was traditionally provided by affordable primary care doctors who actually cared about us and felt a sense of obligation toward us, as we them.

In the next chapter, I will discuss more of how our country has less primary care access and how our mindset helps contribute to this problem.

Moneymaking Medicine

Hospitals these days are one-stop shops. Walking into one is very convenient and easy. My banker did not have time to look for a doctor from her insurance provider handbook, did not have time to make the call, and did not have time to wait for an appointment. She simply walked into a state-of-the-art ER in a hospital near her home.

Hospitals these days are also attractive and convenient places for doctors to refer patients for further workup. My aunt was sent to one within walking distance of her doctor's office for all kinds of available procedures and technologies to diagnose her problem.

The reality is that most medical conditions are minor and can be taken care of by basic care doctors working in primary care offices or urgent care clinics.

The use of attractive, modern-looking hospitals and specialty facilities is a trend in our healthcare market these days. If you enter "hospital expansion" as the search term for news articles in a web search engine, it will return many hits discussing hospital expansions every day. If you walk into emergency rooms or hospitals in your area, you will now see beautifully decorated, comfortable facilities that beat the good old doctors' offices by a mile.

If you know the status of medical practices in your area, you will also know that hospitals and larger healthcare conglomerates, even health insurance companies, are expanding by buying up practices that are struggling financially—basic care doctors and specialists. The recent economic downturn and recent healthcare changes have forced these basic care and specialty practices to join hospitals and larger employers of healthcare providers, such as conglomerates.

What is the purpose and plan for such expansions and for such convenient, beautiful one-stop-shop facilities? That is right—to attract more foot traffic and to generate more revenue. Patients with minor medical conditions who walk into such facilities are guaranteed to incur expensive medical bills, whether necessary or not.

Why do you think this practice of overprescribing medical procedures continues without any legal recourse? The answer is *because it can*. It is simply because medical practices and medical providers can order any procedures they want and can claim the payments for them no matter their reasons for ordering them—whether to prevent lawsuits or to generate more revenue—even if they are ordered without any medical indication. As long as these procedures are performed, they are entitled to be paid. Health insurers can try to deny the payments for these procedures all they want, but the bottom line is that there is no law preventing hospitals and medical practices from getting paid when they perform procedures simply to make more revenue, even if they exceed a reasonable standard of care.

Where does this lead to? That's right—more medical bills that are expensive and unnecessary being sent to health insurance companies for processing and payment. This could only mean one thing—an increase in health insurance premiums.

I will explain in Chapter 3 how the transformation from independent practices to consolidated networks of aggressive medical facilities, i.e. healthcare conglomerates, took place and how it has increased the costs of our medical care and insurance premiums.

Profit-Driven Health Insurance

Many people blame hospitals, medical facilities, and even regular medical clinics for our broken healthcare system, while others blame our private health insurance companies.

Health insurance companies, especially before Obamacare was passed, have the best moneymaking business model in our free enterprise economy. What could be better than receiving cash upfront on a regular prepaid basis; having the ability to raise prices and profit margins with little or no federal or state resistance; and being able to keep that cash on hand longer, by employing various payment tactics, in order to use the cash to earn more in investments?

Many of us working in doctor offices and hospitals know how costly and cumbersome it is to bill health insurers in order to get paid, and how difficult it is to be paid adequately. This is because health insurance companies use various tactics to delay or deny payments, optimizing their profits. There are also various tactics used on patients, as well, to help maximize profits.

Many of us patients have considered how advantageous it is financially for health insurers when they increase our copays and force us to buy into a health plan with a high deductible. Rather than money coming out of their pockets (which is from our paid premiums) to pay our medical bills, we end up paying more up-front in the form of higher copays, as well as more on the back end in the form of higher deductibles. The Obamacare mandate will force us to buy even higher deductible health plans because these plans are more affordable than lower deductible plans. Ultimately it means that we have to pay medical bills out of pocket, up to $12,700 per year per family (the maximum out-of-pocked limit allowed by the new law), before our health insurers even start paying.

In addition, legislation has enabled insurance companies to be the best money-making machines in America by granting them a special legal privilege for decades. We live in a free enterprise country where we believe that free and fair competition should be at the heart of all business. This holds true for most industries except for the insurance industry. The McCarran-Ferguson Act, passed in 1945, grants special exemption from federal antitrust laws to all insurance companies and shifts regulatory responsibility to each state. This means that it is legal for insurance companies to monopolize their market as long as they do not interfere with each state's insurance regulations. This exemption explains why in many states, there is only one major provider of health insurance in the private sector. One example is Blue Cross that dominates more than 83% of the markets in Alabama and almost 80% in Hawaii, Maine, and Rhode Island, according to the report, "Health Care Competition: Insurance Market Domination Leads to Fewer Choices," published by the Center for American Progress in June 2009.

As a result, instead of having hundreds of large health insurance companies competing with one another and offering us competitive health insurance premium prices, we have fewer than ten giant health insurers that dominate the private healthcare system.

What Is the True Underlying Cause?

Is it fair to say that medical practices and health insurance companies are the main causes of our broken healthcare system? Definitely not. And this book is not saying that they are, otherwise the solution would logically be to avoid medical practices, hospitals, and health insurance. That's not really an option for many people now, is it?

We need our doctors. We need our hospitals. And we need our health insurance. This book is not here to point fingers. This book is about

- helping us understand the problems in our healthcare system;
- helping us identify the root cause of these problems; and
- helping us derive the right solutions and necessary actions.

Medical practices and health insurance companies, in and of themselves, are not the causes of our broken healthcare—it is the dysfunctional interaction between the two entities that has led to the most fundamental problems in our healthcare system: high medical care costs, high cost of insurance premiums, and not enough primary care access to keep us healthy. Therefore the true cause of our broken healthcare system and its three fundamental problems is *the system itself* along with the transformation in the past that has allowed such a dysfunctional interaction between healthcare providers and health insurance companies to exist. I am particularly talking about the ability of medical practices to get paid for procedures they order no matter the reasons, and the lack of competition among health insurance carriers as the result of antitrust exemption.

Moreover, the problems in our declining system will now be augmented by further inevitable transformation brought about by the Obamacare mandate unless all of us embrace the complementary solutions suggested in later chapters of this book. If we continue to lack regulation on what medical practices can order and get paid for and lack pricing competition among health insurance plans, further transformation will only worsen the problems we have. Both problems of high medical care costs and high premiums will only get worse once the Obamacare mandate takes effect in 2014 for individuals and 2015 for employers when it mandates that people and employers buy health insurance and forces health insurers to cover people with preexisting medical conditions (which should have been the case from day one).

Once purchased, people with preexisting medical problems will flock to doctors, ERs, and hospitals for long-needed procedures. Medical practices, which already look for more procedures, will generate more claims to health insurance plans when seeing these patients who finally have coverage.

Medical care bills and health insurance premiums will significantly and quickly increase starting in 2014, mirroring the premium increases in the state of Massachusetts after the Massachusetts mandate took effect in 2006, making Massachusetts the state with the highest insurance premiums in 2011, according to The Commonwealth Fund in December 2012, as shown in Illustration 2 below.

Dollars

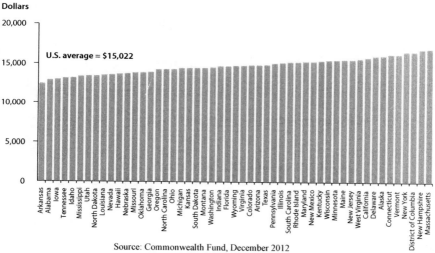

Source: Commonwealth Fund, December 2012

Illustration 2. A graph showing the premiums for family coverage by state in 2011 with Massachusetts being the highest while Arkansas remains the lowest.

The real question we should ask is How can medical care costs come down as long as hospitals and medical practices can be paid for procedures they order solely to increase revenue? For example, why should an MRI ordered for back pain, due to simple muscle sprain, be paid when it is not medically indicated? We are now seeing MRIs ordered for patients with simple back sprains and these bills are getting paid, even though the use of the MRI exceeds a reasonable standard of care (i.e., an anti-inflammatory or muscle relaxant medication and physical therapy for one week). The point here is that our system rewards the escalation of medical care costs. Not only that, but the current trend of hospital expansion by acquisition—buying up smaller medical practices and creating awesome convenient one-stop medical facilities—is positioning health providers to do even more unnecessary procedures and to generate even more revenue. The end result is no ceiling on how far insurance premiums can rise.

Many of us are relieved that Obamacare is finally limiting the profit margin of health insurers to 20% of their premium income (and 15% of premium income from groups of more than 100 full-time employees). Finally! But despite this profit margin limitation, premiums are not prevented from rising. Premiums will continue to rise proportionally at 20% or 15% above medical care costs without a ceiling to cap off both the medical care costs and the insurance premiums, as demonstrated in Illustration 3, below. This is why Obamacare alone will not repair our broken system—it limits health insurance profit margins but fails to limit what doctors, hospitals, and conglomerates can do to increase medical costs and associated health insurance premiums.

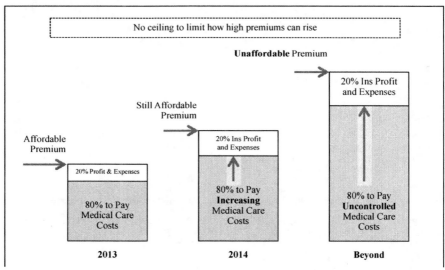

Illustration 3. A demonstration of how health insurance premiums will keep on rising infinitely because: 1) medical care costs can rise without limits, and 2) there is no ceiling to cap off the insurance premiums, despite the inability for health insurance companies to make more than 20% in profit margin.

One can imagine that the ability of premiums to rise infinitely will reach a tipping point where insurance funds are unable to pay for medical care costs because it becomes cheaper for individuals and employers to elect to pay the penalties and not buy health insurance to contribute to the funds.

The system that our health insurance companies and our medical practices operate within is clearly the true cause of our healthcare problems. I will shine more light on this in Chapter 5.

Additional help and action by all of us in conjunction with Obamacare during this transition is becoming the only true solution.

"No Worries Houston, We have a Solution"

Do you ever wonder why your car insurance premium is never as high as your health insurance premium? Do you ever let your mechanic bill your car insurance for engine repair or oil changes? Imagine that our car insurance were used to pay for any car maintenance or expected repairs—wouldn't our mechanics be tempted to do all that they could, including unnecessary repairs, so they could bill our car insurance and generate more revenue? Also, wouldn't we bring in our cars more often to get our premiums' worth in repairs? Were that the case, our premiums would rise, inevitably and rapidly. That's why car insurance is for unexpected losses only, and that's the key to keeping premiums down.

There are more than 250 million registered vehicles in our country. If car insurance companies were paying for oil changes and engine repairs for these 250 million cars on top of what they are paying now for collisions, there would be no way for them to stay in business charging their current rates. They would have to raise their premiums just like our health insurance carriers do in order to survive and be profitable.

If we want our health insurance premiums to be lower, just like that of our car insurance, we will have to avoid using health insurance plans to cover "everything" such as regular maintenance and expected medical care. If we hope to enjoy lower health insurance premiums, then we must use health insurance to cover only unexpected care resulting from major accidents, illnesses, or catastrophes. Unlike car insurance, our health insurance cost is high because it covers checkups, maintenance of chronic diseases, and expected minor illnesses and injuries. It does this for millions of insured consumers, on top of covering care for unexpected, costly major medical events such as heart attacks, cancer, organ transplants, etc.

Therefore the obvious solution for bringing down health insurance premiums is to separate coverage for expected expenses from unexpected losses. Patients can pay expenses for expected care directly to their medical providers while leaving the payment for unexpected medical emergencies to health insurance plans. When the third party is removed from the expected care picture, the potential for abusive overcharging and overprescribing that currently affects both consumers and insurance companies will significantly decrease. Afterward, if a doctor continues to impose exorbitant charges and unnecessary procedures on patients directly, the patients will just leave the doctor for a competitor, leaving the doctor with less business. Paying for expected care directly to doctors without health plan involvement would potentially result in less use of unnecessary procedures. It would also increase competition among providers to provide superior care at more competitive prices.

The next step is to identify what kinds of affordable, direct-pay programs basic care providers and specialists can come up with to make this work. This is what our free enterprise system is all about—the generation of competition and creating high-quality products and services at affordable prices.

Look at the competitiveness of oil changing stations like Jiffy Lube, Grease Monkey, and others. They are competitive in price and quality of service. They have to lower their prices to compete with one another to please customers who pay them directly. They take excellent care of my car with promptness and friendliness when I use them. The same should apply to providing preventive basic medical care and even specialty medicine.

The expenses for unexpected losses and major medical needs can then be taken care of by health insurance companies. The cost of covering unexpected medical loss is greater per visit or per incident, making it harder for an individual to pay. At the same time, the likelihood of such unexpected losses occurring is low enough, when compared to 100% of all insured needing expected care, for insurance to cover effectively. Therefore, in order to lower insurance premiums, major medical catastrophes such as surgery for appendicitis or care of a heart attack should be paid for by health insurance, while leaving the smaller expenses for us to take care of. The combination of paying for small stuff ourselves and leaving major medical costs for our health insurance will result in an overall reduction in costs and premiums.

Chapters 6 and 7 will demonstrate how all of us can work together with our doctors to collectively create an affordable and accessible direct-payment solution to cover expected medical care, one that costs much less than covering it through our health insurance. Again, in doing so we leave the insurance funds to cover major unexpected costs we cannot afford to cover ourselves. This will, in part, help transform our healthcare system from its broken state into a healthy state—the healthcare revolution we need.

Who Will Make It Happen?

Our healthcare system, along with Obamacare, lacks two important keys that are necessary to prevent its demise. The two missing keys are
1. cost control of medical care and procedures that will prevent insurance premiums from skyrocketing; and
2. competition among health plans that will force them to provide more competitive prices.

In other words, unnecessary medical care and procedures push insurance premiums proportionally upwards, while there is no competition to help cap or bring down the rising premiums. However, we can make these two objectives happen ourselves. Then you may ask how we will step up and make these two key changes happen, and what engine will we use to make such difficult changes take place?

Believe it or not, *the answer lies within us.* The answer also lies in our history, going back to 1929. The history of our healthcare started on the right foot at that time—we prepaid our doctors and hospitals directly. But soon thereafter, a smart businessman quickly stepped in and changed the process of prepaying the doctors directly to prepaying the middleman, giving birth to our modern idea of "health insurance," with Blue Cross being the first, albeit nonprofit, health insurance company.

Unlike car insurance, health insurance took off in the wrong direction by starting to cover both expected care and unexpected losses (basic care and advanced care) from the beginning. Covering both has not led to crisis until now, when the costs of the care and the premiums to cover those costs are becoming unaffordable.

We simply cannot wait for anyone else to come in and rescue our private healthcare system. We must take control of the situation as consumers by using the same method that was used before that middleman stepped in and created health insurance in 1929—by prepaying our doctors for expected care. If we do this, we will reestablish a caring relationship with our doctors, become healthier overall, and visit ERs and hospitals less. Soon, health insurance premiums will have to come down. We can prevent the demise of private sector healthcare. Chapter 7 will discuss how in detail, but we will preview it briefly here.

The engine I use in my clinics is simple and hardly innovative because it was discovered in 1929 in Elk City, Oklahoma by Dr. Michael Shadid. The engine is the prepaid "medical membership" model, the same concept as our current health insurance model but one wherein doctors are prepaid directly, bypassing the health insurance middlemen. The medical membership model, with its more affordable prices and strong doctor-patient relationships, will reduce our healthcare costs by preventing excessive and unnecessary medical procedures. This addresses the first missing key—cost control of medical care. It will then automatically help create the second missing key, the creation of competition in a new area of healthcare as well as in the insurance market, which will help bring down insurance premiums further.

We simply need to go back to prepaying our doctors and our specialists for taking care of our chronic problems, minor illnesses, minor injuries, and regular checkups. We can urge our doctors to make it available in their practices. Then we both participate in creating and sustaining this cost-saving prepaid system for expected medical care. When we and our doctors work together, the two most desirable objectives will finally be met:

1. Our doctors will become independent of control by healthcare conglomerates, hospitals, and health insurance companies.
2. Doctor-patient relationships will be reestablished to help keep us healthy and out of hospitals, emergency rooms, and operating rooms.

In doing so, we leave our health insurance funds available to cover just unexpected, costly major medical problems, thereby avoiding depletion health insurance funds or growth in insurance premiums.

The Ideal Healthcare Picture—Is it Realistic?

On an individual scale, imagine my aunt calling her doctor for the Bell's Palsy symptoms and imagine the doctor being independent of a healthcare conglomerate, so he does not feel obligated to drive up the bills to generate revenue. Imagine that my banker had a similar doctor, one with whom she was happy, so she could leave ER visits to patients needing advanced and true emergency medical care. At the same time, my aunt and my banker both continue to have their health insurance plans available in the event of catastrophic medical need, but at a much lower premium because their direct prepaid medical membership programs keep them healthier and generate no medical claims for their health insurance companies to pay out. Then, imagine renewing their health plans the following year with a decrease in premium—which has never happened before in our healthcare history.

On a much larger scale, imagine a healthcare system where free enterprise principles are put into correct use again and our private healthcare system remains intact without total governmental control. There is an extensive nationwide network of private medical membership programs competing with one another, offering the best preventive health programs at the most competitive prices for basic care and maintenance of chronic problems. At the same time, our current private health insurance companies remain in the market and continue to offer coverage for medical catastrophes just like a true insurance carrier should, but with much lower premiums. The combination of both plans fulfills the Affordable Care Act requirements and mandate. Our hospitals and their lifesaving facilities continue to provide major medical care and receive their payments from private health insurance companies for major medical procedures. They will not have to deal with a total government-controlled healthcare system with challenges similar to those of Medicaid and Medicare, because private health insurance companies remain healthy in our system.

TWO

CHAPTER 2
Underuse of Basic Care Medicine

There is no doubt to many that the most important type of physician in the US healthcare system is the good old family doctor. This chapter discusses how patients are not utilizing this affordable healthcare resource and the reasons why. It demonstrates one reason why our system is transforming into one that has higher healthcare costs.

The Traditional US Medical Model

Healthcare providers and facilities in our country can be divided into two broad categories: basic and advanced. It is important for everyone to distinguish basic healthcare from advanced healthcare and to understand the pricing associated with the two.

Basic healthcare providers are family doctors, internal medicine doctors, and pediatricians, collectively called "primary care" physicians. These providers are responsible for continuously taking care of general health problems and regular checkups for adults and children, i.e. basic care medicine. Their facilities generally are basic medical offices and walk-in clinics that often do not have high lease expenses. They do not have expensive advanced medical equipment. They employ basic medical receptionists and medical assistants who are not costly to hire. They also do not offer expensive procedures such as ultrasounds, CT scans, or MRI scans. Urgent care clinics are also considered basic care providers.

Basic care providers also diagnose and treat minor illnesses and injuries, in addition to taking care of chronic medical problems. Most of the time, a basic care doctor can make a diagnosis and give treatment by just using the two most basic tools in medicine—their stethoscopes and their prescription pads. Some patients will need additional diagnostic procedures and treatment. These are basic procedures that can be easily performed in their clinics. They include rapid strep tests, urinalysis, pregnancy tests, x-rays, splinting, casting, giving shots, and basic breathing treatments—none of which are costly to provide in a doctor's office. For example, a rapid strep test costs only $1.51 per test. These basic medical procedures, when necessarily performed, help reduce healthcare costs by preventing patients from getting worse and ending up in ERs, hospitals, or specialty clinics.

Advanced healthcare providers, on the other hand, are specialists who have training beyond that of basic healthcare providers. They help care for medical conditions too advanced to be handled by basic care providers, such as heart attack, appendicitis, deliveries, and complications from chronic medical problems. Examples of such advanced care providers are general surgeons and specialized surgeons, orthopedists, cardiologists, obstetricians, gastroenterologists, endocrinologists, and emergency room physicians. Most of them are set up in advanced healthcare facilities such as emergency rooms, hospitals, surgical centers, specialist hospitals, and specialist clinics—which are all more costly to operate and maintain than basic care facilities. This is due to higher operating and build out costs and the need to have advanced medical equipment and specialized medical personnel to care for the patients.

Advanced medical care can be much more expensive when compared to basic medical care. It includes costly diagnostic and therapeutic procedures such as endoscopy, surgery, CT scans, MRI scans, cardiac catheterizations, and much more. Often these advanced procedures are performed in hospitals or in surgical centers so their fees end up having two components, a professional fee (charged by the doctor) and a facility fee (charged by the hospital).

In a traditional medical model, a community is typically served by a local hospital that has an emergency room, operating rooms, and nursing units with patient beds to take care of patients admitted to that hospital. Family doctors, internists, and pediatricians usually have their offices located close to the hospital in the same community. The combination of the hospital (advanced facility) and medical clinics (basic facilities) makes up the dynamic of a healthcare network for that community. It is traditional for patients to see their primary care doctors first for any medical problems, as opposed to walking into an ER (emergency room) right away. Patients visit their basic care providers for regular care of chronic diseases such as diabetes, hypertension, and heart disease, for checkups, as well as for any acute illnesses or injuries, such as sore throat, cough, or lacerations.

First, family doctors do their best to workup medical problems, making a diagnosis and providing a treatment, and then refer patients to specialists or hospitals only if necessary when further workups are required. This stepwise approach to medical issues is the traditional model of medicine. Another important component that follows this traditional model is that after seeing their patients, the doctors then bill their patients' health insurance for payment because most patients have health insurance coverage.

This traditional model of accessing primary care doctors first is now fading as our healthcare system goes through a transformation, resulting in less basic care access and usage, and more usage of advanced, state-of-the-art facilities. Additionally, there are increasing financial and ownership connections among healthcare providers—that is, healthcare conglomerates are increasing in number and size.

My aunt's case is a good example of a traditional model gone wrong. She was initially taken care of by her primary care doctor, but then quickly and unnecessarily referred to a state-of-the-art emergency room to receive specialized care for a condition that was benign, basic, and self-resolving. Her experience is one of millions that contribute to the overuse of emergency rooms with their exorbitant costs. Her $16,000 emergency room bill is a small fraction of the billions of dollars wasted in emergency room use each year.

Why Has the Traditional Model Changed?

More people have been turning to emergency rooms (ERs) for their basic healthcare for the past several decades. This shift from visiting regular physicians to visiting emergency rooms started in the 1950s. It marks the beginning of a major shift away from using traditional doctors for basic medical care needs first. According the *Western Journal of Medicine*, there were 18 million ER visits in 1958. This number increased to 77 million visits in 1977. The source further disclosed that as many as 70% to 85% of such visits were for non-urgent problems.

Emergency department (ED) visits in the United States increased 28% between 1992 and 2005, according to a publication by Dr. Ellen J. Weber from the Division of Emergency Medicine at the UCSF School of Medicine as published in the *Annals of Emergency Medicine* in 2008. The Henry J. Kaiser Family Foundation also published a statistic showing that in 2010 there were anywhere from 268 to 712 ED visits per 1,000 population in each of the 50 states, Hawaii being the lowest and District of Columbia being the highest.

According to the New England Healthcare Institute (NEHI), the number of *non-urgent* ED visits increased dramatically from 9.2 million in 1997 to 16 million (nearly 14% of total ED visits) in 2005. This overuse is responsible for at least *$38 billion dollars* in wasteful healthcare spending each year. NEHI president Wendy Everett, ScD, said that non-urgent ED overuse is not mainly due to use by the uninsured, as is widely believed. She claimed that "non-urgent ED use is increasing in tandem among all payer groups, including those covered by both privately and publicly sponsored insurance." There are several attractive reasons for the increasing overuse of emergency rooms. They offer several benefits, including:

- Convenient 24-hour access.
- A wide range of services.
- Widespread insurance acceptance.
- Immediate reassurance for patients' medical conditions.
- A legal obligation to treat all walk-in patients.

These are some technical reasons for ER overuse, but they do not explain all of the reasons that contribute to the degeneration of the doctor-patient relationship, as well as the skyrocketing price of healthcare.

I have learned, through my 15 years of experience in talking to patients and treating them in my urgent care clinics, especially in recent years, that there are three main reasons why they end up going to ERs over basic care physicians. These reasons are reflected in three attitudes that many people have about healthcare in our modern era. These attitudes have resulted in private primary care doctors becoming underutilized, and people ending up in advanced care facilities such as emergency rooms, hospitals, and specialist clinics. The three most prevalent attitudes include:

- "I cannot afford to see a doctor, so I will wait."
- "I won't see a doctor until I have health coverage."
- "I don't have a doctor" or "I cannot get in to see one."

"I Cannot Afford to See a Doctor, So I Will Wait"

Many people hold the mindset that since healthcare is expensive "I won't go to a doctor until I absolutely have to." The general public has expressed more unrest concerning the costs of healthcare, even those with health insurance. I gather this knowledge from being exposed to the patients in my clinics, who tell my staff and me that they delay seeking help because of cost. Both the insured and uninsured tell me the same thing, where the insured are paying a copayment (copay) of $20 to $40 and the uninsured are paying a $119 flat fee in my clinics.

For example, the doctors in my clinics see patients with full-blown pneumonia who should have come in to be treated earlier when the condition was still a sinus infection that had not yet gone to the lungs. We would then end up treating these patients with a daily antibiotic shot (in order to see improvement faster, prevent complications, and minimize economic loss by avoiding a hospital stay) until the patients are much better while allowing them to finish their treatment with an oral antibiotic. Often they don't come in for their follow-up appointment the next day as instructed—again because of costs—only to end up returning a few days later because the pneumonia had not gone away or had worsened.

According to the *2012 Commonwealth Fund Biennial Health Insurance Survey* in April 2013, roughly 80 million people—around 43% of America's working-age adults—did not go to the doctor or access other medical services in 2012 because of cost. This is up from 75 million people two years ago and 63 million in 2003. The hesitation to visit doctors is due to the increase in copays and deductibles that often makes patients responsible for the entire bill.

To many people, a $20 to $40 copay is a lot because it competes with paying a telephone bill or other necessity. Ironically, some of these same people will often pay $80 to $120 for a haircut and hair coloring, making the cost of a copay seem trivial. Taking care of one's health for a low price in order to avoid an exorbitant cost from ER or hospital bills should be at the forefront of everyone's mind if we want our nation to be healthy with a lower cost of medical care. Compared to specialist care, the price for basic medical care by a general practitioner is low and much more affordable for both the insured and uninsured in the long run.

Payments to basic care doctors from health insurance plans are also not high. If you have Medicaid or Medicare, their payment for a family doctor visit is state dependent, but can be as low as $50 and $70, respectively. (The Affordable Care Act now makes payments for Medicaid and Medicare the same.) If you are insured, private insurance will reimburse from $60 to $200 per visit with a copay from $20 to $40 for a family doctor.

People think that medical care costs are high perhaps because they fail to distinguish between basic and advanced healthcare. So they mistakenly believe all medical care is prohibitively expensive. In reality, basic medical care is not expensive and therefore cost should not be a deterrent to the general public.

I wish I had had a chance to interview the healthy 35-year-old patient described in the first chapter who died needlessly of probable streptococcal sepsis. I would ask him why he waited so long to see a doctor for his sinus and throat problems. He probably held the same general view the public has about healthcare—it costs too much. Had he understood the low cost of basic care and sought early treatment, his death could have been prevented.

Furthermore, if we take the insurance billing component out of this traditional model, the cost of seeing basic care doctors becomes even more affordable which is contrary to what the public believes. In other words, if the middleman is removed from the picture and patients pay their doctors directly (as opposed to billing their insurance and end up with a balance due to a deductible), basic medical care becomes a lot cheaper as illustrated by the table on page 118.

For example, if you are uninsured and need periodic basic care at an affordable price, you will want to visit a general practitioner like Dr. Vern Cherewatenko in Bellevue, Washington and pay cash for his care. His patients are happy that he is their primary care doctor because they pay only $50 cash for each visit. His entire office is as small as a typical clinic's waiting room. In a CBS News interview Chuck O'Brien, a 55-year-old self-employed patient, described Dr. Cherewatenko's practice this way: "This is traditional medicine. This is what America was like thirty years ago. It is a whole world of difference."

Another example of an affordable cash clinic is the 5 Minute Clinic located in Heber City, Utah. Owned by Elmer Sisneros, a physician assistant for twenty years, this cash clinic charges only $65 per visit. Even patients with high-deductible insurance plans find that it is much cheaper to visit Elmer's clinic and pay cash than go through their insurance for claim processing.

"I Won't See a Doctor Until I Have Health Insurance"

The second mindset that negatively affects and weakens the traditional model of medicine is the idea that insurance coverage is needed before seeing a doctor.

Frequently I come across friends and family who ask for medical advice in casual conversations. Sometimes I am shocked when they describe symptoms of an advanced state of disease, and I tell them, "You need to see a doctor." They often reply, "I can't afford to see a doctor until I have health insurance." This is either because they believe they will be exploited by a doctor if they don't have health insurance, or they truly believe their insurance will cover "everything."

First, the public needs to know that traditionally basic care providers, such as family doctors, internists, and pediatricians are trained to be cost-conscious in their practices. Most do not perform a lot of procedures, and they try to keep the costs down. Training programs for primary care doctors typically teach them to rely on history taking and examination skills to diagnose problems, as opposed to performing expensive diagnostic procedures.

Despite the trend to join hospitals and the push toward procedure-based medicine, many basic care providers are fighting to stay in private practice. They stay with traditional medicine and continue to rely on their clinical skills to diagnose and treat without ordering a lot of expensive procedures. Many of them have decided to convert their practices to cash only in order to stay in private practice and offer affordable medicine.

Second, the public needs to also know that most health insurance these days may not "cover everything" after a copay is paid. Until recently the public truly believed that health insurance coverage is an absolute must and could be counted to cover everything once a need arises. Wendell Potter, in his book *Deadly Spin*, reveals that he was paid well for almost two decades by two large health insurance companies to make Americans believe that they cannot live without health insurance. Many Americans have had the idea instilled in their heads by insurance advertising campaigns that the modern rendition of health insurance is a necessary part of their lives, consequently too many Americans buy a health insurance policy and expect it to cover all of their medical care costs.

Misperceptions about the necessity or coverage offered by most health plans leads more and more people to delay seeing doctors. They often wait until they find an "affordable" health insurance policy, thinking that once this health insurance is in place, they will not have to pay much for medical care. The reality is that between high copays and high deductibles, even the insured are paying more than they can comfortably afford for healthcare.

What more and more people are discovering is that after paying several hundred dollars in monthly insurance premiums, a visit to a doctor or a healthcare facility often results in the entire balance being the responsibility of the patient. A lot of insurance plans have now "cost-shifted" to their members in the form of high deductibles, higher copays, or other hidden costs that patients are held responsible for. These health insurance plans are also providing less and less in coverage, only to result in higher patient out-of-pocket balances. The purpose of these higher-deductible plans is to make the premiums affordable and make the consumers think twice before incurring costs. Thinking twice and hesitating to seek care, as discussed earlier, can work against patient health—an unfortunate trend.

In February 2013, the *Annals of Family Medicine* conducted a study on out-of-pocket cost sharing for healthcare expenses and their social, medical, and financial disruptions. The study found that high levels of cost sharing cause considerable anxiety, substantial debt problems, threat to non-medical household budgets, as well as disruptions to medical care. Here are some of the quotes from the study's participants:

- "I couldn't take it. I can't afford it. The copay was even too hard to handle.... I said, you know what, I'd rather be sick."
- "It's scary because when you know you've had colon cancer ... and you know that every month you put off [going to the doctor] ... you're hurting yourself."
- "[I] wouldn't go to the doctor unless I just could not stand ... the pain."
- "... it's going to get harder.... We have really great credit. I hate to ruin that, but it looks like it might get ruined if we can't afford to pay all these high medical bills."
- "... I couldn't heat the house."

Finally, once purchased and in place, one would hope that a person would take their health insurance and rush to see a family doctor for a regular checkup or health screening to prevent major illnesses. Paradoxically, this is not the trend. From what I see in my clinics, insured people still tend to put off seeing their doctors until urgent medical needs arise. When a need does arise and escalates into a serious illness, a person may not have a familiar family doctor to access and will likely and conveniently walk into an emergency room or hospital.

"I Don't Have a Doctor" or "I Cannot Get in to See One"

The third reason our traditional healthcare model is undergoing a transformation is an increasing nationwide shortage of basic care providers. Many patients use my urgent care clinics over the years because they say, "You guys are my primary care doctor." They will frequently say, "I cannot get in to see my doctor," or "I don't have a primary care doctor, so I always use your urgent care clinics." This mindset reflects the shortage of primary care physicians in this country.

Policymakers are increasingly realizing that there is a nationwide shortage of primary care providers who are a necessary part of improving our nation's health and controlling our healthcare costs. Despite this awareness, the shortage of primary care physicians is worsening without improvement in sight.

According to the National Association of Community Health Centers in March 2009, 56 million Americans, or nearly one in five, lack adequate access to primary care due to a shortage of primary care physicians in their communities. This is the result of a decline in the primary care workforce. Poor reimbursement to primary care physicians from insurance carriers, lower income than other types of physicians, and a poor quality of work life are among the major reasons fewer doctors are choosing to become primary care physicians.

Allen Horn, President of CentraCare Clinic of CentraCare Health, a health system in Minnesota, stated, "The number of family medicine trained US medical student graduates has decreased more than 50% in the past five years. In internal medicine, those who specialize in adult and geriatric medicine, less than 2% of medical students are going into office-based internal medicine." These office-based internal medicine practices are key to keeping adults and the elderly, with chronic medical problems, healthy—a number that is growing vastly every year, including 70 million baby boomers who are accessing Medicare as of 2011.

One reason for the shortage of primary care doctors is that medical students are not choosing to become primary care doctors and are choosing specialty fields. Today only 35% of physicians are basic care providers versus 50% in the mid-1950s. Lower career earnings in the primary care field, when compared to specialty fields, is the main reason for this decrease. For example, the 2011 Review of Physician Recruiting Incentives by Merritt Hawkins shows that the average salary for a family practice physician is $178,000 when compared to $355,000 for an anesthesiologist and $402,000 for a radiologist. There's little wonder why new doctors are not going into primary care fields.

According to a white paper survey conducted on behalf of the Physician

Foundation in October 2010, there are other factors that discourage graduates from becoming primary care doctors. Primary care doctors have a less desirable lifestyle because they are ultimately caring for the whole health of their patients on a chronic basis and are often required to be available for their patients 24/7 by health insurance companies with whom they have contracts. Compare this to specialists who take care of patients belonging to primary care doctors only when needed. Primary care doctors have long hours, receive less reimbursement, and have to deal with more paperwork and extra administrative tasks without extra compensation. Fewer than 30% of current primary care physicians surveyed indicated that they would choose primary care if they had to choose their career again.

Weak Doctor-Patient Relationship

The traditional model of medicine that I am referring to in this chapter involves accessing medical care via primary care physicians first (who are cost conscious and are not usually influenced by other entities simply to generate profits) as opposed to walking into ERs, specialist clinics, or hospitals as the first point of access. A major component of this model, of course, is a strong relationship between patients and their primary care physicians in private practices. This is the model that we are moving away from in the US healthcare system in recent years. With fewer and fewer independent primary care doctors, there is no doubt that doctor-patient relationships in this country will further deteriorate. The result is an increase in healthcare spending and a higher mortality rate when compared to other countries that have easier access to primary care medicine.

According to a *British Medical Journal* (BMJ) article published in November of 2003, the United States ranked 16th out of 19 countries on mortality from causes amenable to healthcare (excluding ischemic heart disease), where the death rate was 81 persons out of 100,000 from ages 0 to 74. On the same scale, countries with open access to healthcare, especially primary care, had lower death rates, such as Sweden (51 out of 100,000), Norway (57 out of 100,000), and Australia (61 out of 100,000).

Over the years, fewer and fewer people feel they have a working relationship with a primary care physician. Decreasing numbers of primary care doctors and people's perception that basic healthcare is prohibitively expensive are not helping to improve this relationship. Higher copays and higher deductibles make it even worse. Without a strong bond between primary care doctors and patients, medical care costs will be difficult to control and will rise steadily—accelerating the demise of the American healthcare system as we know it.

In the past, people had personal family doctors who took care of them since birth. First, obstetricians delivered babies. Then the babies were passed on to pediatricians or family doctors to care for, performing well-baby checks, giving proper vaccinations, and caring for any illnesses during the childhood years. As adolescents and adults, people consulted with the same family doctors who knew them well enough to assist with prevention, so basic medical problems were taken care of sooner and at a lower cost. This is because the long-term relationship allowed the patients to call their family doctors for advice, or just go in for a quick visit with little or no social or financial hesitation. This type of trusting association is fading in America.

In the past, there was little hesitation for family doctors to give consultation over the phone without having to see their patients or run confirmatory tests. This was considered a reasonable standard of care in a long-term, well-developed doctor-patient relationship. Doctors also did not hesitate to call medications in to the pharmacy without seeing the patients first because of the trusting relationship and the known medical history. Such relationships created less fear for malpractice litigation and allowed low-cost medicine to be possible in the past. The practice of treating over the phone or treating without having to do many tests does not exist much these days in private practices, due to the risk of malpractice and the need to generate revenue. So patients frequently come into my urgent care clinics because their doctors could not just call in their medications and do not have same-day appointments available for them.

Had Karen, my banker discussed in the first chapter, been seeing a family doctor on a regular basis for her yearly checkup as well as for her existing illnesses, she could have just called, walked into her doctor clinic, and be seen for her kidney stone without much cost incurred.

These days, healthy adolescents and adults typically become "lost in the system" for reasons such as: being healthy and not seeking preventive care; switching health insurance carriers; and having busy lives with less time for preventative measures until medical needs arise. The practice of maintaining a relationship with a family doctor is even much harder and less attractive nowadays when everyone thinks that going to the doctor is too expensive. As a result, many healthy people, as well as increasing numbers of unhealthy ones, decrease their doctor visits until they have problems or until their problems worsen, at which time they conveniently walk into emergency rooms for help.

In my clinics, as well as in various social settings, I see many people go on with their lives without family doctors until suddenly they have medical problems or until they turn 40 to 50 years old. Many live their lives without annual checkups to screen for medical problems in order to take care of them early to avoid escalation of these problems. Then when major medical issues occur, what follows is a sudden panic and scramble to seek medical help and a trusting doctor-patient relationship that can only be developed over time.

Institutionalization of Physicians

There is another factor that has facilitated further deterioration of the private doctor-patient relationship. In the past, primary care doctors did not have much difficulty running their practices, so they could take care of their patients with full autonomy. In the past few years, however, they have been struggling to stay afloat economically because of the increasing costs of running a practice.

While many new medical school graduates these days do not prefer to become primary care physicians—causing a nationwide shortage—it is also perfect timing for existing primary care practices nationwide to sell their practices to hospitals or join healthcare conglomerates. This merger and acquisition activity has been quite extensive for the past few years in the Salt Lake City area led by three large companies that own local hospitals and medical practices. They have been acquiring both primary care practices and specialty practices, including family doctors, internal medicine doctors, cardiologists, orthopedic surgeons, and even neurosurgeons. What is the risk posted by such acquisitions? That's right, the potential of a push toward overutilization of advanced, state-of-the-art hospitals and specialty facilities, as opposed to cost-saving, individual private relationships between doctors and patients.

It is becoming difficult these days for primary care doctors to sustain their private practices within the traditional model of seeing patients first, billing their insurance, and then getting paid a few months later. The overhead for such a single-doctor clinic is anywhere from $30,000 to $50,000 per month. If the average insurance reimbursement for a patient visit is $100 per visit and the overhead is $40,000 per month, for example, a primary care doctor will need to see about 18 patients a day, working 8 hours a day and 5 days a week, just to cover the practice's overhead expenses. At 18 patients a day, each patient will receive about 30 minutes per visit, which is generally adequate time to establish a healthcare relationship. Of course if insurance carriers pay less than $100 per visit—for example Medicaid which pays about $50 per visit (before Obamacare took effect) and Medicare which pays about $80 per visit—the doctor will need to see more than 18 patients a day.

However, keep in mind that in this scenario of seeing the patients first and then billing their insurance for payments, 18 patients per day will only cover costs. To make the practice profitable where the net income (before tax) is equal to an average annual salary of $150,000 for a family doctor, the doctor has to see 6 more patients per day, working 5 days a week and being reimbursed at $100 per visit. The patient load now becomes 24 visits per day. This allows the primary care doctor to spend only 15 to 20 minutes per patient. This might be adequate time for a follow-up visit, but not for a new patient, and especially not for internal medicine patients who frequently have multiple medical problems, and who ideally require up to one hour or more for the initial visit. This is at $100 per visit. For Medicaid and Medicare patients who pay less than $100 per visit, the doctor will have to see more than 24 patients per day to sustain his practice. It is a no wonder that many physician practices are dropping Medicaid and Medicare patients.

A reader may stop here and note that Dr. Vern Cherewatenko in Bellevue, Washington (who charges $50 per patient per visit) and Elmer Sisneros, PA in Heber City, Utah (who charges $65 per patient per visit)—both mentioned earlier—have no problem making a profit in their practices. The reason is that these two are a type of provider that is not the same as the typical doctors that I am discussing for the most part, because they bypass insurance billing that's slow to pay—*by months*. These two providers are paid cash right away at the time of service. This emphasizes the cost burden brought about by insurance billing. It is seen as a major overhead cost and delay in payment that must be avoided in order to remain solvent for these doctors.

Upon interviewing a local hospital executive, I was informed that most of the primary care practices that get bought out are still in the red financially, even after joining hospitals. Hospitals continue to support them only because they recoup their losses and make a profit from the hospital referrals these practices make. Is it any wonder that fewer and fewer medical students are choosing to become primary care physicians, and that more and more of the existing primary care physicians are closing their private practices?

The *Accenture Physicians Alignment Survey 2012* reported that independent physicians continue to dwindle and that those remaining are increasingly becoming employed by health conglomerates or hospital systems, resulting in a drop of independent physicians from 57% in 2000 to 39% in 2012. By the end of 2013, Accenture estimates that independent physicians will comprise only 36% of the market.

As an example of practice takeover, recently St. Luke's Health System in Idaho rapidly bought physician practices, from general practitioners to cardiologists to orthopedic surgeons. About 1,400 doctors in southwestern Idaho are now employed by St. Luke's or its smaller competitor, Saint Alphonsus Health System.

According to *American Medical News*, 21 physician practice mergers and acquisitions occurred in the second quarter of 2012, with $4.2 billion changing hands. "You're going to be seeing more hospitals buying physician practices to control referral sources and to have a better and bigger say in quality as they start to get penalized for readmissions," said Stephen M. Monroe, editor of *Health Care M&A Report*.

It is becoming uncommon these days to see newly graduated primary care doctors, or even specialists, start their own practices from ground zero. They will usually either join a large private practice or join practices owned and operated by hospitals where the first one to two years of salary is guaranteed. *American Medical News*, in October 2011, reported that graduating residents are now seeking employment from hospitals rather than starting their own practices or joining private ones. A survey of these residents by Merritt Hawkins & Associates reported that 32% of residents in 2011 preferred to join a hospital-based practice over a private practice, a significant increase from 3% back in 2001. They reported the top five worries for these residents to be:

- Availability of free time
- Billing issues
- Inadequate income
- Malpractice expenses
- Healthcare reform

All of these worries exist above and beyond the debt they incurred in medical school.

The End Picture

As the result of decreased access to primary care and increasing utilization of ERs since the 1950s, the US healthcare system is the most costly in the world. Nations with easy access to primary care, such as Japan, Canada, and the 10 members of the European Union (EU), have lower healthcare costs and lower mortality rates. The Commonwealth Fund, whose purpose is to promote a high performance healthcare system, explained that few patients in Denmark, England, France, Germany, the Netherlands, and Sweden reported unmet needs for care or found general care unaffordable.

The *OECD Health Data 2011* compared spending on healthcare in the United States with spending on healthcare in other countries from 1980 to 2009, and found that the United States spends more on healthcare per capita than any other country. See Exhibit 1.

The same *OECD Health Data 2011* also reported that none of the 12 selected countries spent more than 12% of gross domestic product (GDP) on healthcare, compared with 17.4% by the United States, which is $7,960 per capita, as shown in Exhibit 2.

In summary, people are hesitating to see their primary care doctors

Exhibit 1. International Comparison of Spending on Health,1980–2009

Average spending on health
per capita ($US PPP)

Total expenditures on health
as percent of GDP

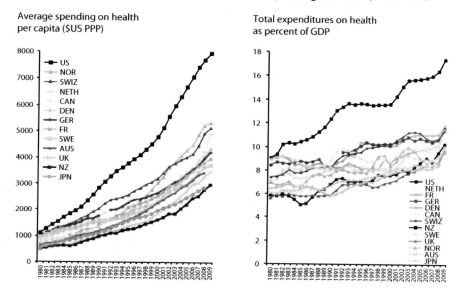

Note: PPP = Purchasing power parity—an estimate of the exchange rate required to equalize the purchasing
power of different currencies, given the prices of goods and services in the countries concerned.
Source: OECD Health Data 2011 (Nov. 2011).

Exhibit 1. International Comparison of Spending on Health from 1980—2009. The first graph clearly
shows that the United States has the highest average spending on healthcare per capita since 1980. The
second graph also shows that the United States has the highest total expenditure on healthcare as a percentage of gross domestic product (GDP) since 1980. Both graphs clearly show that we are the world
leader in healthcare spending.

because they either don't have health insurance or their copays and
deductibles are higher, causing more out-of-pocket expenses. Many of these
patients end up becoming sicker and less healthy, requiring visits to ERs,
hospitals, and specialists when they finally decide to seek help. Shortages
of new primary care physicians and institutionalization of physicians and
their practices increase the trend of visiting ERs and hospitals even more.
Hospitals and healthcare conglomerates see this opportunity and expand
their facilities, adding specialists and procedures, and then acquiring even
more primary care practices to help attract patients in order to increase
referrals for these specialists and procedures. This results in even more overutilization of advanced healthcare providers and procedures, resulting in
the United States being the largest spender of healthcare in the world and
bringing us to a national healthcare crisis.

The Demise of our Healthcare

Exhibit 2. Health Spending in Select OECD Countries, 2009

	Population (millions)	GDP per capita[b]	Total health spending		Health spending, by source of financing		
			Per capita[b]	% GDP	Public	Private	Out-of-pocket
Australia	22.0	$39,924	$3,445 [a]	8.7%[a]	$2,342 [a]	$476 [a]	$627 [a]
Canada	33.4	$38,230	$4,363	11.4%	$3,081	$646	$636
Denmark	5.5	$37,706	$4,348	11.5%	—	—	—
France	62.6	$33,763	$3,978	11.8%	$3,100	$587	$291
Germany	81.9	$36,328	$4,218	11.6%	$3,242	$424	$552
Japan	127.5	$32,431	$2,878 [a]	8.5%[a]	$2,325 [a]	$99 [a]	$454 [a]
Netherlands	16.4	$41,085	$4,914	12.0%	—	—	—
New Zealand	4.3	$28,985	$2,983	10.3%	$2,400	$184	$399
Norway	4.8	$55,730	$5,352	9.6%	$4,501	$43	$808
Sweden	9.3	$37,155	$3,722	10.0%	$3,033	$69	$620
Switzerland	7.7	$45,150	$5,144	11.4%	$3,072	$504	$1,568
United Kingdom	60.9	$35,656	$3,487	9.8%	$2,935	$188	$364
United States	306.7	$45,797	$7,960	17.4%	$3,795	$3,189	$976
OECD Median	10.7	$33,434	$3,182	9.5%	$2,400	$193	$559

[a] 2008.
[b] Adjusted for differences in cost of living.
Source: OECD Health Data 2011 (Nov. 2011).

Exhibit 2. Health Spending in Selected OECD Countries in 2009 showing that the United States has the highest total health spending per capita when compared to all of the countries in this study.

Three

CHAPTER 3
Moneymaking Medicine

This book, as outlined in Chapter 1, argues that we have three major issues in our healthcare system that increase the cost of medical care and health insurance premiums. Chapter 2 discussed the underuse of basic care medicine as the first major issue. It revealed statistics showing the increase in ER usage and some reasons in patients' minds that have contributed to the underuse of basic medicine. It also pointed out how our doctor-patient relationship has diminished and why basic care providers have become employed by larger institutions, as opposed to staying in private practices.

Now this Chapter will discuss the second major issue and how it impacts our healthcare system—aggressive, money-making, state-of-the-art medicine. First I will show how I was personally trained to become a conservative basic care doctor. Then I will demonstrate how, despite the purpose of such training, our system has transformed medical practices and healthcare conglomerates to become financially aggressive, resulting in higher spending in US healthcare. The rest of the chapter will disclose statistics illustrating this problem and show that the quality of care in the United States is not reflected in a positive way by the fact that our healthcare expenses are the highest among 12 other industrialized countries. In other words, the *more* the cost is not necessarily the *better*.

Conservative Medicine—How It Worked in the Past

In my past 15 years as an urgent care physician (since 1998), I have seen my fair share of healthcare changes, but nothing compares to the changes I have seen in the past five years.

I spent my time as a medical student from 1990 to 1994 at the University of South Alabama in Mobile, Alabama. I started my first experience with patient care during my clinical rotations from 1992 and 1993 at the University of South Alabama Medical Center. At that time, I was taught that the best practice of medicine was to make a medical diagnosis and then provide treatment in conservative ways with the goal of cost savings at the forefront. We would depend our diagnostic ability on careful history taking as well as on our examination skills. We based our decisions to diagnose and give treatment on clinical judgment, rather than on the results of advanced (and expensive) diagnostic procedures such as CT and MRI scans. We would see hospitalized patients in the morning and have roundtable discussions on medical workup and treatment plans as a team, led by an attending physician. We would order diagnostic tests or procedures only if necessary and give treatments only if needed, keeping medical care costs in mind. We also would consult with specialists only if necessary. The specialists at the time also relied on their clinical skills and physical exam skills, as opposed to ordering expensive diagnostic procedures at the drop of a hat.

The teaching and practice of conservative medicine continued to be observed during my internal medicine residency years at the University of Utah Medical Center from 1994 to 1997, as well as into my first several years of practice. During my residency years, I was allowed to order consultation from specialists and order diagnostic procedures only if I ran out of options after using my own clinical skills and after discussing the cases with the attending physician and my colleagues in training. The teaching of conservative medicine also applied to outpatient care in clinical settings.

After finishing my residency training, I continued this practice of conserving healthcare costs and healthcare resources in my private practice. I also observed this philosophy being used by other colleagues in their practices in other communities in those earlier years.

In the past our healthcare system embraced conservative and traditional methods of diagnosis and treatment. Most family doctors, internal medicine doctors, pediatricians, and even specialists, practiced under their own private professional corporations with little or no financial ties to each other. The family doctors would have enough time to spend with their patients, working up their patients' medical problems for some time before sending them to specialists for further assessment and care. They would refer patients to specialists only if necessary. Specialists also did not appear to be so eager to see a large volume of patients, nor did they order or perform specialized procedures right away. Back then most of these doctors were in their own practices, earning a decent salary. Most of them were not employed directly by hospitals or by corporations that owned hospitals and other health facilities. Because of this they did not have the incentive to use hospitals excessively and would only use them if necessary and according to a reasonable standard of care.

In the past there was also a much more clear-cut financial separation between physicians and hospital systems, probably because physicians were content with their earnings. This differs markedly from what is going on today where there are increasing numbers of private practices being bought out by hospital chains and healthcare conglomerates to help channel patients to their facilities, resulting in increased use of advanced procedures and treatments.

Dr. Manoj Jain, an infectious disease specialist and writer for the *Washington Post* reported, on March 12, 2012, that increasing numbers of doctors are becoming hospital employees rather than staying in private practices. In his city, a dozen practices totaling more than 100 doctors have been purchased in two years by various hospitals. The Medical Group Management Association also reported that in 2002 about 20% of US physician practices were hospital-owned. This number jumped to over 50% in 2008.

Why Conservative Medicine Is Dying

When encountering difficulties in running their private practices and deciding to sacrifice their independence, most physicians are fortunate enough to find alternate employment in time. Some have to file bankruptcy. According to *CNN Money,* in April of 2013 some physicians were still able to keep practicing after filing bankruptcy but, for others, it's a career-ending event. Bobby Guy, co-chair of the American Bankruptcy Institute's Health Care Committee, noted that Chapter 11 bankruptcy filings by physician practices have spiked recently.

According to *CNN Money*, Dr. Denis Morgan, an oncologist in Enfield, Connecticut finally filed for bankruptcy in June 2011 after struggling to fight shrinking reimbursement for treatments and chemotherapy drugs. His hundreds of chemotherapy patients at the time suffered and had to find alternatives.

Another physician, Dr. Morgan Moor, an internist with a once-striving solo practice in Brentwood, Tennessee, told *CNNMoney* that she lost almost half of her patients by 2010 due to the recession. With a drop in her revenue of nearly 30%, she almost had to file for bankruptcy in 2011. However, she was able to restructure her debt and her business without filing.

While most struggling physicians seek employment with large employers to stay in the medical professions and some file for bankruptcy, a few simply pick up and leave our country. One example is Dr. Grady Snyder who "gave up on health care in America" and moved to Australia and took up rural medicine there. He was a thriving family physician in the rural areas of Pueblo, Colorado for 16 years, taking care of 5,000 patients. A third of Snyder's rural patients were using Medicare, the reimbursement for which started to shrink in the 1990s, causing his revenue to drop while the costs of running his practice kept rising from year to year. The cost of having an electronic medical record system, which became a legal requirement in 2009, was the final straw for him. He had to give up what he loved doing in America, caring for patients he knew well and cared about. He then moved to Australia, and is making the equivalent of US$250,000 a year—$100,000 more than he made practicing medicine in Colorado.

The struggle to stay afloat is not the only problem facing primary care doctors who try to follow conservative medical practices. Other specialists, such as cardiologists, who try to conserve costs by performing procedures in outpatient settings also struggle and have to close their practices due to decreasing reimbursement. A great example is when Medicare reimbursement for outpatient cardiology services started being cut in 2010 by 10% to 40%. At the same time, the reimbursement for the same procedures performed in hospitals, which are normally charged more to begin with, increased even more. For example, Medicare pays a hospital $400 for an echocardiogram and $180 for a cardiac stress test, while it pays $150 and $60, respectively, if performed in a physician's office, according to *Bloomberg* in November 2012. Dr. Thomas Lewandowski, a Wisconsin cardiologist faced with this dilemma, decided to sell his practice to a local hospital and become one of more than 6,000 employees of ThedaCare, which runs five hospitals and many clinics in Wisconsin.

The Need to Stay Viable

A good question to ask is if doctors were trained to practice conservative medicine which is best for our long-term health, why are they not doing everything they can to maintain their traditional belief and practice?

It is a great question because we doctors want to do whatever is right to keep healthcare accessible and affordable. But the answer lies in the system itself and all the changes that force doctors and medical practices to do whatever they have to in order to stay afloat economically. Otherwise, if they maintain their conservative stance, they may end up filing bankruptcy or closing their practices like the doctors discussed above.

As mentioned previously, if a practice relies mainly on insurance billing, then family doctors, internists, and pediatricians would have a difficult time making it financially, seeing only 15 to 20 insured patients per day—they would have to see more. The need to see more patients explains why you will not get doctors to call in prescriptions anymore. Most doctors will require you to go in for a visit even if they know precisely what is wrong and have been prescribing the same medication to you for years. Additionally, you may see more procedures being performed when compared to the past, even by primary care doctors. The reason behind this is also the need to generate more revenue compounded by the need to minimize malpractice potential, which can cause the cost of running a practice to be even higher.

Even when these basic care doctors become employed by hospital networks, their revenue still does not cover the cost for many of their practices. As mentioned before, according to a local hospital executive I met during a meeting, the reason hospitals continue to employ these doctors in their practices, even though they still run in the negative, is because the referrals to their hospitals for procedures and admittance makes it worthwhile financially.

Malpractice Insurance Costs

Another reason you will no longer see your doctor simply calling in prescriptions over the phone, beside their need to generate more revenue from your visit, is so they can minimize malpractice potential. For example, if one of your family members tests positive for strep throat and you start to come down with similar symptoms, your doctor will likely not call in a prescription to treat without seeing you, whereas in the past many of them would. This is because symptoms of strep throat can mimic symptoms of pneumonia. If pneumonia is missed and a wrong antibiotic is called in for treatment and resulting in morbidity and mortality, the doctor can be sued which negatively impacts his credentials and increases his malpractice cost.

Because of our increasingly litigious society, medical malpractice costs have steadily increased across the nation, resulting in more difficulty for doctors to maintain their private practices.

The Cost Is Up

The cost of running a medical practice is higher than in the past. The lease for office space is not as cheap as it used to be. The clinic build-out cost is also much more now, due to higher costs of materials and labor. Payroll costs are higher compared to the past, because of increased cost of living. Medical billing is more difficult and costs more and more each year, due to unpaid accounts and increased compliance requirements. In addition, the mandatory use of electronic medical record systems also incurs extra fees. For billing reasons alone it has become more difficult and very costly for doctors to stay in private practices.

The Pay Is Down and Delayed

The biggest hindrance to maintaining a private practice is that the reimbursement for medical care by health insurance carriers and patients is reduced and increasingly difficult to obtain. Medical practices use their own cash to run their operation. Instead of being paid right away in cash for services rendered, a practice receives credit in the form of account receivables, namely, the amount that the practice is entitled to bill health insurance plans and patients for, not the actual payment itself. In other words, patients receive medical care right away but the payments do not come into the practice until several months later. Therefore each practice must have enough cash in reserve to operate while waiting for these payments to come in. Each medical practice also has to have an in-house billing department or else outsource to a billing company which adds cost, and all of this while following strict and costly billing rules and regulations. Medical billing costs about 8% to 10% of a medical practice's total revenue, on average. As discussed earlier, doctors Morgan, Moor, and Snyder are great examples of doctors with troubled practices due to decreased reimbursement.

Additionally, cost-shifting to patients, in the form of increased copays and higher deductibles, causes medical practices to receive less money for their services. For example, 10 years ago in the early 2000s, patients frequently had no copay, or a $10 to $20 copay for a visit to a family doctor. For a $100 visit, the practice would receive $90 or $80 from the health insurance in one or two months. Nowadays the patient's copay is either higher or the whole visit cost becomes the patient's balance, due to their deductible requirement. The average copay to see a family doctor is now about $30 per visit. In such cases health insurance pays $70 for a $100 visit. This is actually a 22% discount for the health insurance carrier when compared to the $90 it used to pay in the past when the copay was $10. Furthermore, if the patient has a high-deductible health plan and has not met their deductible, then the whole $100 becomes the patient's responsibility, which is a 100% discount for the insurance company and often an insurmountable burden for the patient. Once it becomes the patient's responsibility, the balance usually takes three to six months before it is paid, increasing back-end billing costs. Of the deductible balances due from my patients, only 70% actually get paid, while the remaining 30% get sent to collection due to nonpayment. These numbers are actual numbers from my own practice.

A person who knows nothing about our healthcare system could easily wonder how doctors in our country have allowed themselves to become stuck in a situation where they have to pay cash out of pocket to take care of their patients' health with the hope of being paid by the patients' insurance, but instead have to go after that patient for reimbursement several months down the road. Theoretically, and like the prices of goods and services in other sectors of the economy, medical service prices should logically increase from year to year, thus enabling doctor practices a cost-of-living increase. Instead, health insurance companies' payments to doctors have decreased as the years have gone by, to the point where the insurance companies don't have to pay for doctor visits at all—the patients do, which defeats the purpose of having insurance. With high-deductible health plans, this becomes inevitable.

These are the reasons why family doctors cannot afford to spend much time working-up patients' problems anymore. They need to see more patients per day and spend less time per patient to make their practices viable financially. Today, family doctors who bill insurance plans need to see 25 to 30 patients per day as opposed to 15 to 20 patients like in the past. To achieve such numbers, it has become easier for doctors to spend 10 minutes on each patient and send the patient to specialists for further care and workup or have the patient come back more frequently. By doing so doctors can see three to four patients an hour, allowing them to obtain viable revenue. However, achieving such high number of patients per day is not easy during this recession.

Additionally, unlike the $10 copay of the past that did not discourage patients from visiting their doctors, higher copays and high deductibles now discourage patients from visiting their doctors. This increase in out-of-pocket pay, in turn, causes the volume of patient visits to their doctors to decrease, therefore negatively affecting their business and adding more stress to medical practices nationwide. In September 2008 the *Wall Street Journal* reported that consumers were reducing healthcare spending and that visits to doctors dropped between 2007 and 2008. In one of the studies they looked at, 22% of consumers reported going to the doctor less often. Additionally, The Commonwealth Fund reported in April 2013 that 43% of

America's working-age adults did not go to the doctor in 2012 because of cost.

Many existing practices around the country, therefore, are forced to consolidate with larger employers, hospitals, or healthcare conglomerates if they want to remain viable. Furthermore, if being in private practice is difficult and no longer attractive these days, what do medical graduates do when they come out of post-medical school training? The answer—they are becoming specialists and joining hospitals or large healthcare employers. The era of conservative medicine and private practice is ending and has transformed into an era of aggressive medicine, in which state-of-the-art facilities and procedures are increasingly used with profit as the principle motive, increasing the costs of healthcare astronomically.

So far this chapter has discussed reasons why medical practices are forced to abandon conservative medicine and have transformed our healthcare system to aggressive medicine. The rest of this chapter will demonstrate how this transformation has impacted the cost of healthcare and will show that it has not improved overall health outcomes in the end.

The Transformation to Aggressive Medicine

It has become clearer in the recent years that conservative medicine is transforming into aggressive medicine. In August 2011 the Center for Studying Health System Change published a study stating that hospital employment of physicians has accelerated in recent years to shore up referral bases and capture admissions. Poor reimbursement rates, rising costs of private practice, and a desire to have a better work-life balance have contributed to physician interest in hospital employment. It goes further to say that this trend may increase costs through higher hospital and physician insurance payment rates and hospital pressure on employed physicians to order more expensive care.

In the first year of joining them, hospitals usually guarantee a doctor's salary. Thereafter the doctors' salaries are derived by a revenue-based system called Relative Value Units or RVUs. The RVU system allows the employer to pay less salary if the physician produces less revenue, and more salary if the physician produces more revenue for the hospital or related clinics. RVUs reflect the relative level of time, skill, training, and intensity required of a physician to provide a given service. A simple well-patient visit, for example, would be assigned a lower RVU than a visit that is complex and requires workup procedures. A physician seeing a few complex or high acuity (seriously ill) patients per day could accumulate more RVUs, and therefore a higher salary, than a physician seeing many patients but with less complex problems. Nationwide, increasingly more physicians have their salaries tied to RVUs, being compensated more for seeing patients requiring more procedures. One may say this is a fairer way to compensate a physician for seeing difficult patients. However, in my experience, an RVU system easily opens the door to abuse that causes further increase in our healthcare costs. One of my past colleagues, whom I worked with under a large healthcare employer, would elect to perform additional unnecessary procedures on his patients just to raise the RVU of those patients, which in turn augmented his own salary.

Once employed by a hospital or healthcare conglomerate, physicians gain easier access to the rest of the hospital network and resources, enabling them to conveniently refer their patients to specialists and to use diagnostic tools, therapeutic procedures, and advanced technologies. The RVU process urges physicians to order procedures and make their patient visits more complex thus increasing RVUs and thereby the physician's salary. This easy-to-refer process helps increase the use of the hospital's facilities, equipment, staff, medications, and supplies with one ultimate goal in mind—profit making. One may argue that this process may not be true or may not be as dramatic in nonprofit hospitals. However, nonprofit hospitals have similar operating costs. Physicians in such hospitals are often in the same situation of being pressured to generate the same revenue stream to support the costs of running nonprofit hospitals.

This modern healthcare structure of hospitals and conglomerates hiring physicians provide

1. convenience for medical doctors to care for their patients without restriction;
2. easy one-stop shopping where patients can get everything the doctors order in one place; and

3. more opportunity to perform more procedures and bill health insurance plans for greater revenue.

The emergence of such large healthcare structures results in more revenue generation when compared to specialists and primary care doctors seeing these patients in their community clinics, especially when they have no financial ties to hospitals or to healthcare conglomerates. These larger structures of healthcare providers make hospitals and their affiliated practices more efficient revenue-generating machines.

One point of view that may support this one-stop-shop structure of convenient healthcare providers is that it may be the best demonstration to the world that the United States has state-of-the-art medical facilities designed to save lives and increase longevity. However, such hopeful outcomes are not the case. A study by the OECD, discussed below, does not show that the United States has better healthcare outcomes when compared to other countries.

High Healthcare Spending in the United States

It is no surprise to hear that our country is the top spender in the world when it comes to medical care. One would logically guess that this is likely due to our aging population, our higher incomes, our greater supply or utilization of hospitals and doctors, or even due to our smoking rate. However, this is not the case.

The rest of this chapter will demonstrate that our country is the top spender of medical care in the world and this is due to overtreatment, unnecessarily high prices, and more readily accessible technology; and yet healthcare outcomes are no better—and in some cases worse—than those of other countries. In the previous section I pointed out how easy it is for a doctor to conveniently order procedures within a larger healthcare structure and that the doctor has incentive (via the RVU salary system) to over-order and over-treat. (There is no legal regulation from our government to prohibit the use of unnecessary procedures and being paid for them.) Now the rest of this chapter will discuss how unnecessarily expensive some of these procedures are. These high prices, combined with overtreatment, simply make the United States the country with the highest cost of medical care, as well as not the country with the best care.

According to the World Health Organization (WHO), the United States has the highest healthcare spending in the world, which was 17.9% of its Gross Domestic Product (GDP) in 2011. This number is steadily increasing and is projected to reach 19.5% by 2017. In 2006 the United States spent $2.1 trillion on healthcare, or $7,026 per person. This number increased to $2.7 trillion, or $8,680 per person in 2011. Such per capita spending correlates with health insurance costs rising twice the general inflation rate, according to a report in May 2012 from the Health Care Cost Institute, a Washington group that examined data from insurers. The increase in healthcare spending also accounts for 62% of all bankruptcy filings in the U.S., according to the National Patient Advocate Foundation in a white paper published in September 2012.

Not Due to Other Factors

Using data from the Organization for Economic Cooperation and Development (OECD) published in May 2012, David A. Squires of The Commonwealth Fund issued an analysis comparing US healthcare spending to that of 12 other industrialized countries: Australia, Canada, Denmark, France, Germany, Japan, the Netherlands, New Zealand, Norway, Sweden, Switzerland, and the United Kingdom. He stated that the United States spends far more than any other country in the study. Additionally the analysis revealed that the increase in spending by the United States was not due to having a higher per capita income, having an older population, having more smokers, or having a greater supply or utilization of hospitals and doctors. His findings showed:

1. Only 13% of the US population was older than 65 in 2009, compared to 16% average for all of the 13 countries.
2. Only 16% of the adult US population was a daily smoker when compared to the average of 21.5%.
3. The United States had 2.4 physicians per 1,000 of the population in 2009, fewer than all other countries in the study.

4. The United States had fewer hospital beds per population (2.7 per 1,000), shorter lengths of stay for acute care (5.4 days), and fewer discharges (131 per 1,000)—all less than the average for the studied countries in each of the 3 areas.

Due to Higher Prices

We all know that US medical facilities are full of advanced medical technology, making us the country with the best state-of-the-art medicine in the world. But most of us do not realize that the prices for each procedure resulting from this advanced medical technology can be high or low with a variety of prices in between for the same procedure. In other words, there is a lack of standardization in medical procedure pricing in the United States. This variation is especially obvious when comparing clinic prices to hospital prices for the same tests and procedures.

There is a huge difference in price between care given by doctors inside a hospital setting versus in a private clinic. Take my aunt's case as an example. The first CT scan was performed in another clinic outside of the hospital building before she went into the ER. The cost for the first CT scan was $301. The second CT scan was performed in the hospital and cost $3,101! The MRI performed in the same hospital immediately after that CT scan cost $3,201. That same MRI would have cost less than $700 at a typical outpatient MRI facility. A great example is U.S. MRI in Salt Lake City which charges $500 per MRI study for patients who pay cash.

How can our country control our healthcare costs when there is no standardization of pricing—let alone knowing the prices at the time of service—for various medical procedures? The answer is that we cannot control it. This is why, when compared to other countries, the United States has higher prices for medical care. This includes prices for hospitalization, surgeries, diagnostic imaging studies, and even for seeing primary care doctors and specialists.

David A. Squires, through the same Commonwealth Fund study of May 2012, supports my claim that the costs of medical care are unnecessarily high in the United States. Here are some of his findings:

- Hospital stays in the United States were far more expensive than in the other study countries, exceeding $18,000 per discharge, compared with less than $10,000 in Sweden, Australia, New Zealand, France, and Germany. This spending is three times the median of $6,222 for all the study countries. See Exhibit 1 below. This finding could indicate that US hospital stays tend to be more resource-intensive than in other countries or that the prices for hospital services are higher.
- The prices for the 30 most commonly prescribed drugs are one-third higher than in Canada and Germany, and more than double the price they are available for in Australia, France, Netherlands, and New Zealand.
- Spending on physician services is generally higher than in other countries. For example, primary care physicians generally receive a higher fee for office visits, and orthopedic physicians receive higher fees for hip replacements than in Australia, Canada, France, Germany, and the UK.

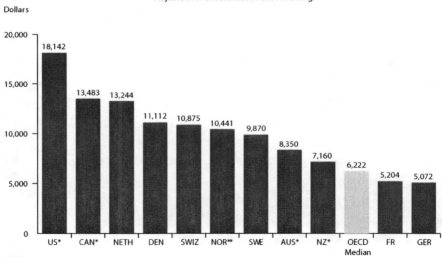

Exhibit 1. Hospital Spending per Discharge, 2009
Adjusted for Differences in Cost of Living

Dollars

* 2008.
** 2007.
Source: OECD Health Data 2011 (Nov. 2011).

The Commonwealth Fund study states that one explanation for high US health spending is the greater use of more expensive medical technology than other countries. The OECD also tracked the supply and utilization of several types of diagnostic imaging devices, which are often costly technologies. A comparison of MRI, CT, and mamogram usage is shown in Exhibit 2 with the following specific findings:

- The United States performed 91.2 MRI exams per 1,000 people (43.0 being the median for all of the countries combined) with an average price of $1,080 per exam.
- CT scans were performed 227.9 times per 1,000 people, far exceeding the median of 122.8 for all the countries. The average CT scan price of $510 per exam in the United States far exceeded other countries' prices of $122 to $319.
- The United States performed 40.2 mammograms per 1,000 people with a median of 17.3 for all the countries.

Exhibit 2. Diagnostic Imaging in Select OECD Countries

	MRI machines			CT scanners			PET scanners	Mammographs
	Devices per million pop., 2009[c]	Exams per 1,000 pop., 2009[c]	MRI scan fees, 2011[d]	Devices per million pop., 2009[c]	Exams per 1,000 pop., 2009[c]	CT scan (head) fees, 2011[d]	Devices per million pop., 2009[c]	Devices per million pop., 2009[c]
Australia	5.9	23.3	—	38.7	93.9	—	1.1	24.3
Canada	8.0	43.0	—	13.9	125.4	$122 [e]	1.1	—
Denmark	15.4	37.8 [a]	—	23.7	83.8 [a]	—	5.6	17.0
France	6.5	55.2	$281	11.1	138.7	$141	0.9	—
Germany	—	—	$599	—	—	$272	—	—
Japan	43.1 [a]	—	—	97.3 [a]	—	—	3.7 [a]	29.7 [a]
Netherlands	11.0	43.9	—	11.3	65.7	—	4.5	—
New Zealand	9.7	—	—	14.6	—	—	0.5	26.4
Switzerland	—	—	$903	32.8	—	$319	3.0	33.2
United Kingdom	5.6 [a]	—	—	7.4a	—	—	—	9.0
United States	25.9 [b]	91.2 [b]	$1,080 [f]	34.3 [b]	227.9 [b]	$510 [f]	3.1 [a]	40.2 [a]
Median (countries shown)	8.9	43.0	—	15.1	122.8	—	1.1	17.3

[a] 2008.
[b] 2007.
[c] Source: OECD Health Data 2011 (Nov. 2011).
[d] Source: International Federation of Health Plans, 2011 Comparative Price Report: Medical and Hospital Fees by Country (London: IFHP 2011).
[e] Nova Scotia only.
[f] U.S. commercial average.

Overtreatment

There is no doubt that a good portion of medical care in our country is from overtreatment and overuse of procedures. In December 2011, Dr. Donald Berwick, the Administrator of the Centers for Medicare &

Medicaid Services, stated that 20% to 30% of medical care is a waste, listing overtreatment of patients as one of the five causes of the waste. He cited other causes which include
- suboptimal coordination of care;
- administrative complexity of the healthcare system;
- burdensome rules; and
- fraud.

Many of us, whether we are patients, healthcare providers, or the general public, have personally encountered overuse of healthcare resources at some point in our lives, either on ourselves or on family members or friends. My aunt's case of Bell's palsy is always going to be a great example of overuse and overtreatment. To reiterate, she did not really need a repeat of the CT scan. The radiologist or the ER doctor should have reviewed the first CT scan before the second CT scan was ordered. Then the second CT scan result should have been reviewed before rolling her into an MRI scan, which was performed immediately without a good reason. Additionally, the expensive IV medications and the expensive lab draws could have been held off pending the results of the scans, especially when the presentation was quite obvious for Bell's palsy rather than a bleeding stroke. Lastly, a portable chest x-ray was performed. The x-ray was absolutely unnecessary for her condition of Bell's Palsy and was not indicated for a hemorrhagic stroke, and it cost $423.30.

No Improvement in Outcomes

Despite the high costs and increased usage of advanced medical technology, the quality of care and the outcomes of the US healthcare system are not necessarily better than the far less expensive systems in the other study countries, according to the same OECD study.

Studying a various array of healthcare quality indicators, David A. Squires from the same Commonwealth Fund analysis also shows that the United States had the best five-year survival rates for breast cancer when compared to other countries, but not for cervical and colorectal cancers. As for the rates of potentially preventable mortality due to asthma (for those between ages of 5 and 39) and lower-extremity amputation due to diabetes per 100,000 of the population, the United States had among the highest rates of mortality and amputation. This suggests a failure to effectively manage asthma and diabetes, two common chronic conditions in the United States.

The rates of in-hospital deaths, among people admitted for heart attacks and strokes within 30 days of admission, were also measured. The US performance for these measures fell in the middle range, not significantly worse nor significantly better than the median rates of death from heart attack and stroke when compared to other study nations.

Certainly one must argue that specialized procedures performed in hospitals are necessary to treating various medical conditions when indicated. One can also argue that even though these procedures are expensive, our total healthcare costs would not be so high were these procedures performed only when absolutely necessary and then reimbursed appropriately. The problem of high healthcare costs arises when these expensive procedures are ordered and performed unnecessarily to generate revenue or defensively to prevent malpractice claims.

For-Profit and Nonprofit Hospitals

One may also argue that only for-profit hospitals exhibit such aggressive and unnecessary utilization of their resources. Sadly, it's not true. There are two types of hospitals: for-profit and nonprofit. For-profit hospitals answer to investors, not to the communities they serve. Their profits go to investors and not back into the community. They are usually owned by companies that are publicly traded. Nonprofit hospitals, on the other hand, give their profits back to their communities by investing in research, new technology, new services, and programs to best meet the healthcare needs of their communities. Based on their charitable purposes, and often affiliated with a religious denomination, they are the traditional means of delivering medical care in the United States. They also get their funding from government grants, foundations, and even wealthy private citizens.

Without regard to their profit status, all hospital administrators are driven by the same bottom line because they all have high expenses they must meet—although either will do whatever it takes to keep the operation going, for-profit hospitals usually have more expenses than the nonprofits. When nonprofit hospitals become cash-poor, they will often seek investors from for-profit firms to keep the hospitals going for their communities. An example of this is the Detroit Medical Center and its network of eight hospitals that were acquired consecutively by Columbia in 2010, then Vanguard Health Systems, and most recently by Tenet Healthcare Corporation in October 2013. Tenet now operates 77 acute care hospitals, 173 outpatient centers, 5 health plans, and 6 accountable care organizations.

For-profit hospitals are increasingly expanding their facilities to increase the traffic of patients. A Google search on "hospital expansion" will return abundant news of hospitals expanding and adding on services every day. Hospitals are modernizing their facilities, making them look impressive and attractive for patients. They are adding services by employing specialists as well as specialized equipment.

One would think that such expansion of both for-profit and nonprofit hospitals would improve health outcomes. Again, and just like the OECD analysis by David A. Squires, such is not the case. In June 2004 the *Canadian Medical Association Journal* published a study by Dr. PJ Devereaux of McMaster University and his team who performed a large-scale meta-analysis on 23 academic papers examining more than 26,000 hospitals. They examined mortality rates and payments for care at private for-profit hospitals versus nonprofit hospitals. Since private for-profit hospitals do not exist in Canada, the research examined US for-profit hospitals. The research shows that for-profit hospitals had 19% higher costs and 2% higher mortality rates. The researchers attribute higher costs directly to the necessity to generate revenue to satisfy investors, administrative costs, and to large executive bonuses. Many believe this focus on profit inevitably led to decreased focus on patient outcomes.

Hospitals and their affiliated network of medical providers and facilities have become better money-making machines in our healthcare industry in the recent years. Nationwide, hospitals are expanding their facilities and provider networks as fast as they can to attract more patients when the Obamacare mandate comes online in 2014 for individuals and 2015 for employers.

Obamacare supporters may argue that more affiliated networks of medical providers and facilities are necessary to the success of Accountable Care Organizations (ACOs) as set forth in Obamacare. The objective of ACOs is to keep Americans healthier by rewarding primary care physicians financially for achieving desirable outcomes. But as long as insurers retain fee-for-service payment method (getting paid for procedures performed), rather than the capitation method (limited pay no matter how many procedures are performed, which will be discussed extensively in Chapter 8), then healthcare costs will continue to rise with no end in sight.

Why All the Changes? It's All About the Money

The dynamic among hospitals, medical clinics, and both basic healthcare providers and advanced healthcare providers has certainly changed from little or no financial connection among one another to a whole new mesh of interrelated networks nationwide. These networks are influenced by the financial interests of all involved with various goals in sight—the biggest one of them being revenue generation.

The overtreatment of patients will only worsen as the consolidation of doctor practices, health facilities, and hospitals increases. If this trend continues, the future healthcare provider structure in our country will consist of networks of healthcare conglomerates employing medical providers, with increasing incentive and focus on channeling their patients toward their own clinics, facilities, and hospitals.

Then there will be increasing numbers of claims sent to health insurance companies as hospitals gear toward increasing their revenues by expanding and buying up medical practices. This can ultimately only mean one thing—increasing health insurance payouts for these claims that will in turn result in higher insurance premiums, higher copays, and higher deductibles.

The next chapter will discuss the role of health insurance companies and how they are the third problem in our private healthcare system. Their continued high profitability will come at the expense of patients and healthcare providers.

Four

CHAPTER 4
Profit-Driven Health Insurance

For a long time many people, including myself, thought that our private health insurance companies were the root cause of our healthcare crisis. But after three years of research, I can see that health insurance companies are only part of the problem (one of three, two of which have been discussed thus far). This chapter discusses facts and insurance tactics that make many people believe that insurance companies are responsible for the current healthcare crisis. Such simplified thinking causes us to miss the real cause of our crisis, leading us to fix only part of our problem as opposed to fixing the entire cause. The next chapter, Chapter 5, will help us discover the root cause of our healthcare problems, one we've been building toward in these first four chapters. But first we must gain a better understanding of health insurance companies and how they work.

The Best Moneymaking Machine in America

Our private healthcare system is all about making money. It is not just medical practices and hospitals that are profit-driven, but also the insurers who collect our premiums and pay our medical bills. The health insurance business has probably one of the best moneymaking business models in our country, one that has been so exploitive in the past that Obamacare targets its profit margins specifically. What could be better than someone paying you money up front monthly that you can put into savings and investment accounts to earn interest? You then delay paying any money out, keeping it in your accounts as long as possible, allowing you to earn yet more interest. You also have a good chance that the people you should pay may forget to follow up on their invoices. On top of all these advantages, you don't have to manufacture any goods and you don't have to provide any services yourself—it's all just administrative work.

To top it all off, insurance companies are exempted from the federal antitrust laws by the The McCarran–Ferguson Act of 1945. This results in the domination of our national markets by fewer than ten large health insurance companies. For instance, Blue Cross is the only major player available in the state of Alabama. There are other states in which Blue Cross is the only major provider. In fact there are 38 Blue Cross and Blue Shield plans nationwide that dominate many markets, including South Carolina, North Carolina, and Virginia. Plaintiffs in North Carolina even filed a major lawsuit against Blue Cross and Blue Shield of North Carolina (that has more than $1.8 billion in reserve), alleging that the insurer drove up health care costs by colluding to carve up the nation's insurance market and illegally agreeing not to compete on one another's turf, according to a report posted on *Charlotteobserver.com* dated February 8, 2013.

Like other multi-billion-dollar businesses, insurance companies contribute significantly to the financial well-being of our economy and the US financial system. Many believe so. In addition to covering expensive medical care costs, they keep our economy healthy, right? Or are they one of the major problems in our broken healthcare system?

Insurance in the Past

In the past, not only were primary care physicians and specialists content to practice private medicine, but patients were also satisfied when their health insurance premiums were affordable. There was little or no out-of-pocket expense, and their healthcare needs were met. The cost of seeing a primary care doctor was not a concern to patients because their insurance coverage paid all expenses with little or no deductible. Because health plans rarely had deductibles, medical practitioners were often paid right away rather than having to turn around and bill the patients.

Patients received better care from their family doctors and specialists because they could spend more time with them and not be rushed through their visits. If the patients were hospitalized, their family doctors were likely to be the ones who took care of them while in the hospital. The family doctor would order tests, procedures, and provide treatment if necessary. They were conscious about cost control and did not have financial incentive for ordering unneeded procedures and treatments, especially hospital-based procedures. Patients' health insurance usually took care of most, if not all, charges incurred in hospitals and the majority of charges incurred for visits to doctors. And most of all, their premiums were affordable.

The good old days of health insurance taking care of medical bills and saving lives at affordable costs are slipping away. We are now playing a whole new ball game.

Health Plans Today

Mike P. worked part-time in one of my clinics as an x-ray technician. In order to meet his expenses and to afford health insurance, he had to work in my clinic as his third job. Through his full-time employer, he paid $400 a month for his family health insurance plan that had a $5,000 annual deductible. His full-time employer paid $625 for the rest of the monthly premium ($12,300 total per year). One year his wife became pregnant and gave birth via normal delivery. After processing all of the medical claims, his hospital and doctor bills came out to be just shy of $5,000. Because of the $5,000 deductible on his plan, his health insurance paid nothing for the medical bills. Mike ended up paying the entire hospital bills and all of the doctor bills out of pocket. None of the $12,300 that he and his employer had paid in premium was used to cover his expenses. By the end of that year, Mike had paid almost $10,000 altogether: $4,800 for the premiums (not including his employer portion) and just shy of $5,000 in medical bills to welcome the new addition to his family.

He stated that his health insurance had never paid for any of his family's medical claims during the normal years either because claims for regular visits to his doctor never added up to the $5,000 deductible. In the year that he needed help the most because of a major medical event (the pregnancy), his health insurance was useless. He wondered what the point of having health insurance was. Where did his money go? The bottom line is that Mike had to pay almost $5,000 extra to have a baby, while his health insurance pocketed over $12,300 in annual premiums from Mike and his employer.

This is just one example in millions. If American families and employers pay so much money to health insurance companies to help cover their medical bills and avoid financial ruin, why is bankruptcy due to medical bills in this country increasing? According to the *American Journal of Medicine* in August 2009, 62.1% of a random national sample of 2,314 filed bankruptcies in 2007 was due to medical bills, with 92% of the debtors having medical debt over $5,000. This 62.1% is up from 46.2%, the number from a study by the Department of Medicine of Cambridge Hospital/Harvard Medical School in 2001. According to another Harvard study examining the state of Massachusetts after its 2006 healthcare law mandated that residents buy health insurance, the actual number of medical bankruptcy filings in the state rose from 7,504 in 2007 to 10,093 in 2009, representing 52.9% of all the bankruptcies filed that year.

Why was medical burden the number-one cause of bankruptcy in Massachusetts during the time when the state claims 97% of its population had health insurance coverage? Furthermore, if the purpose of health insurance is to pay medical claims, why are medical practices, especially basic family doctors, not getting paid enough to stay in business? Why do they end up joining hospitals and healthcare conglomerates?

It's All About Profit

Health Care for America Now, an association representing 30 million people that promote, defend, and improve the Affordable Care Act, released a report in February 2010 showing that the five biggest for-profit health insurers—UnitedHealth Group, Inc., WellPoint Inc., Aetna Inc., Humana Inc., and Cigna Corp.—earned a combined profit of $12.2 billion in 2009, an increase of $4.4 billion or 56% from 2008. In light of this increase in profit, consider that these companies ensured 2.7 million *fewer* people than the year before.

As reported by *amednews.com* on May 19, 2008, during a conference with analysts in 2008, Angela Braly, WellPoint CEO, said "We will not sacrifice profitability for membership." The company then went on to post a record profit of $4.75 billion for 2009, an increase of $2.3 billion or 91%, from 2008. The Indianapolis-based company that operates for-profit Blue Cross franchises in 14 states, ended the year with 1.38 million fewer members, or 3.9% less than the year before.

According to the same source and posted by Emily Berry on April 15, 2011, Aetna CFO Joseph Zubretsky told Credit Suisse investment analyst Charles Boorady on July 27, 2011 that, "We would like to have both profit and growth, but if you have to choose between one or the other, you take margin and profit and you sacrifice the growth line." He was speaking during Aetna's second-quarter conference call.

From such accounts it is clear that the primary goal of these two health insurance companies, at least in the eyes of these executives, was not the health of the people they were called upon to insure. Their first priority was to make a profit for shareholders.

Health Insurance Tactics and Effects on Patients

Health insurance companies have various ways to lower their costs and increase their profits. They earn more revenue by charging high premiums. Then they effectively keep their cost down by avoiding the sale of their plans to people with medical problems in the individual market (which will no longer be legal in 2014 due to Obamacare). They have also shifted medical costs to their members in the forms of higher copays and higher deductibles.

Preexisting Conditions

The best method of making money in the insurance industry is selling insurance plans to those who likely will not use the plan—just like selling life insurance to young healthy people or selling car insurance to older drivers with clean driving histories. The same techniques have been used by health insurance companies for decades, selling insurance to the healthy people and denying coverage to people with medical problems.

Obamacare will allow this practice to continue only until 2014. Until then, health insurers will cover people with preexisting medical problems only through employer-sponsored plans (i.e., group insurance) and not through individual plans. Selling health plans to a large group of people in a business is more profitable than selling to individuals. This is because a large employee groups include many people without medical problems (who pay but likely do not use, whereas an individual often buys health insurance to address health issues. Therefore a group of employees, many of them healthy, have a lower percentage of health plan usage (or simply "usage,") allowing the health plan to earn more premium income with less usage when compared to individuals who buy the same health plan with guaranteed usage. This discriminatory practice has created a confusing picture, causing people to question the true purpose of health insurance.

Nevertheless, for the longest time health insurance companies have enjoyed this profitable situation by not having to sell their plans to individuals with existing medical problems. The practice went as far as denying coverage or inflating rates for people who had ordinary medical problems, such as a history of visiting doctors for bladder infections or head colds, according to discussions with various patients in my practice.

Obamacare mandates that health insurers offer coverage to individuals with preexisting conditions beginning in 2014. This may be a win for the nearly 50 million uninsured individuals in this country. Nonetheless, premiums in the individual market will increase significantly to meet the expenses of the sick ones from 2014 onward if insurance companies are to keep their profit margin. The government subsidies help, but are results of tax increases.

Charge High Premiums

In his book, *Deadly Spin*, Wendell Potter, a former lead public relations person for Cigna, speaks of how he had performed his duty well during his 17 years with Cigna in making the public believe that health insurance was a necessary part of life. Many decades ago, health insurance premiums were not a topic of everyday conversation. They were reasonable enough in price as to be unnoticeable. Over the past decades, however, premiums have steadily increased while health insurance campaigns continue to impress the importance of having health insurance in case of medical catastrophe that could cause death or financial crisis. This commitment by the public to continue buying health insurance continued in the past five years despite double-digit percentage increases in premiums, some as much as 49%. Suddenly the public now wonders how it has allowed these insurance companies to charge increasingly higher premiums that are often equivalent to rent or a house payment even though most people seldom use their policies. It is as if we are all frogs in a pan of warm water—the heat is turned up slowly to boil the water, but the temperature rise is so incremental that we fail to realize we are being cooked.

According to The Commonwealth Fund report released in December 2012, the average annual health insurance premium from 2003 to 2011 rose 62% from $9,249 to $15,022, rising significantly faster than income (which rose only 11% for low- and middle-income families during the same period). The average employee premium contribution for a family plan increased 74% from $2,283 to $3,962 in the same period. If this rate continues, family premiums will reach $24,740 by 2020, says the report.

Finally, after all these decades of enjoying large profit margins, the ability of health insurance companies to set their prices to achieve maximum profit margins will no longer be allowed. For the first time in US healthcare history, President Obama was able to pass a law that limits the profit margins and operating expenses of health plans to be within 20% of their premium incomes (15% for incomes from companies with more than 100 employees). The rest of the fund from the premium incomes must be spent on medical care or be refunded back to the insured.

Nonetheless, premiums will continue to rise as long as medical practices can order unnecessary procedures and get paid for them, that is, as long as medical care costs rise, the cost of premiums will rise proportionally despite the profit margin limitation. Premiums will also rise significantly in 2014 and thereafter when insurers have to sell their plans to individuals with preexisting conditions, especially if many employer and individuals elect to pay the penalties and not purchase health insurance plans.

Higher Copays

The rise in health insurance premiums automatically forces people to buy health plans with higher copays because they're more affordable. In doing so, we are automatically allowing our health insurers to utilize an effective tactic in decreasing the insurance payout—cost-shifting to patients. The insurer is able to pay less by making each member pay a little bit more for each doctor visit. A small bump in a copay from $10 to $20 may not seem like much, or be significant enough to discourage a person from buying health insurance, yet this small amount translates to millions of dollars insurance companies do not have to pay out, and therefore increases their profit. If one million patients pay $20 instead of $10 per visit to their doctors in one month, we are talking about that insurance company not having to pay $10 million to the doctors. It is a very effective savings plan for the insurance company. This practice has been so effective at increasing profits for insurance companies that most peoples' copays have gone from $10 in the early '80s to $20 in the '90s to $30 in 2000s, to $40 in the last few years. If this doesn't make us all frogs in a pan of boiling water, I don't know what does.

Most private health insurers seem to mean well by increasing reimbursement of procedure codes by 3% annually. However, if you consider the 22% discount in their payment as a result of increasing the copay from $20 to $30 or from $30 to $40, this 3% annual payout increase to doctors is comparatively little. Imagine an even higher copay that is as high as $75 or $100 per visit to an urgent care clinic whose final bills are five to ten times less than a visit to an ER for the same presentation. This is becoming standard and there is no other justification for it but profit making by insurance companies. Supporters of such increases in copays may argue that this method will prevent people from driving up healthcare costs who frivolously run to their doctors for simple, unnecessary complaints. I see the opposite. Patients are now waiting to come in until they are really sick, causing them to miss more work, need more procedures, and need referrals to hospitals and specialists for further care—all driving up costs rather than saving costs.

Higher Deductibles

Similarly, higher premiums for plans that typically had good coverage in the past have forced many people to buy health plans with higher deductibles to keep their premiums affordable. This is simply insurer cost shifting. In the '90s health insurance plans with deductibles higher than $500 per year were rare. In the early 2000s health plans with deductibles as high as $1,000 per year were few and far between. The popularity of purchasing higher deductible plans did not significantly rise until the mid- to late-2000s because premiums started to increase by double digits from 2007 on. According to The Commonwealth Fund report of December 2012, deductibles more than doubled from 2003 to 2011, increasing an average of 117% per average single-person during the 8-year period. In 2011, 78% of employees faced an increase in deductible, up from 52% in 2003. In recent years health insurance premiums have increased dramatically, making it increasingly unaffordable for individuals to purchase health benefits and for small business owners to offer them. Affordability has been exacerbated by the recession, and now many people have ended up with health plans with $2,000 to $10,000 deductibles, even those with group insurance offered by larger employers.

Health insurance companies, as anyone can suspect, hugely benefit from selling health plans that have an annual deductible higher than $1,000. This is largely due to the following two factors:

    1. An average person visits a doctor about three times per year (1,969 primary care doctor visits and 1,121 specialist visits, annually, per 1,000 population according to actuary data from a large Utah health insurance brokerage company); hence, the average person will not go to the doctor often enough to reach the $1,000 deductible mark for the health insurance plan to start paying.

    2. Eighty percent of most people's medical needs can be taken care of

a by a basic care provider, such as a family doctor, pediatrician, internal medicine doctor or urgent care facility; hence, the payout by insurance for these average consumers significantly decreases, because the insured are forced to pay first, such as the case of Mike P. discussed earlier.

Let's do the math. The average range of cost (reimbursed by private health insurances, not Medicaid or Medicare) for a basic visit to a family doctor is anywhere between $100 to $150 per visit. Let's use four as our average number of visits that a person makes to a doctor in a year's time. The cost for the four doctor visits is $400 to $600. In other words, it would take more than 8 to 10 visits to a basic care provider per year before the health insurance started paying for the doctor visits if the health plan has a $1,000 deductible. Imagine deductibles of $2,000 and more. If you are healthy, you will likely never use your family doctor enough to reach that deductible— just as in the case of my employee Mike who paid out $12,000 in one year's premium (together with his employer) for a $5,000 deductible plan, and whose insurance never paid a dime for the birth of his baby.

This is why some people prefer to drop health insurance altogether, save their money, and pay cash for basic doctor visits. Some who retain coverage do so by purchasing $10,000 deductible plans just in case of major catastrophe.

Are High-deductible plans Really the Solution?

Supporters of health insurance companies may argue that increasing the copays and the deductibles is the best way to prevent excessive use by the insured, and therefore will lower our healthcare costs. Moreover, the Obamacare mandate, just like the Massachusetts mandate in 2006, will force even more consumers to purchase high-copay and high-deductible plans because of their affordability. One would think that this would prevent excessive and unnecessary care, but the opposite is true, based on what I see in the communities I serve. Higher copays and deductibles result in sicker people who end up incurring more medical care costs over the long run, further inflating health insurance premiums. Additionally, medical practices experience less patient volume and end up joining hospitals and other conglomerates who drive up procedures and costs. So, contrary to what supporters of high-deductible plans believe, the problem is not due to the overuse of medical facilities by consumers, but due to the coverage of "everything" and to the overuse of expensive, unnecessary medical procedures by medical practitioners, especially those associated with healthcare conglomerates geared to produce higher profits.

When more insurance money becomes available under the Obamacare mandate, medical practices will want it. Private practices have to get more to survive and to profit. And it's easy enough to get it—just do more and bill more. With the number of advanced procedures available in today's world, it is easy to see how healthcare conglomerates can seize the money in the insurance pot far more easily than private practices because they offer a full spectrum of services. What happens when unnecessary medical procedures get paid without restriction? That is right—medical care costs go up which in turn drive up insurance premiums. Then the mandate drives people to buy the most affordable plans—the high-deductible plans. When insureds access medical care with these plans, they end up footing the entire bill. In this way the state of Massachusetts had the second highest cost per capita personal healthcare spending (at $9,278 per person per year) in the country in 2009, according to the Centers for Medicare & Medicaid Services. It also had the highest insurance premiums in the country at $16,953 per family in 2011, compared to the national average of $15,022, according to a study released by The Commonwealth Fund in December 2012. To top it all off, the Harvard study discussed earlier found that medical bankruptcy filed in Massachusetts rose 34.5% from 2007 to 2009.

Everyone is left wondering what will happen to the rest of the country in the many years to come with Obamacare reform.

Health Insurance Tactics and Effects on Physicians

So far in this chapter I have examined strategies used by health insurance companies to maximize profit from members. Now I will turn to strategies they use against physicians and medical practices to further increase their profit margins.

Delayed Payments

In addition to the cost-shifting to patients, health insurers also utilize various tactics with medical practices to further maximize their profits. One common tactic is simply delaying payments. In General, as we all know, delaying or forgetting to pay our bills allows us to have more money in our pockets for a longer period of time. When health insurers delay paying medical claims, they retain millions of dollars in their bank accounts longer, which gain interest whether they have good reasons for the delay or not.

According to a survey by the American Medical Association in 2004, more than 82% of state medical societies cited delayed payments as the most significant issue facing their members. The California Healthcare Association alone reported that its hospital members were owed nearly $1 billion in claims that were longer than 60 days past due. Many physicians face significant cash-flow problems that forced them to expend substantial resources pursuing unpaid and underpaid claims, according to James W. Marks, reporting in the *Journal of Medical Practice Management* in its November/December 2004 issue.

Most doctors are not savvy about handling finances or running a business. I am admittedly a perfect example of that. During the first several years of my practice, starting in 2000, I never paid attention to my billing and collection processes in detail. I never paid attention to what was paid and what was not paid and the reasons behind them. When I started to pay attention to that department, I audited past claims and discovered a high number of claims with delayed payments. Most of these claims would have been ignored and not paid at all had my billers not performed follow-up calls to insurance companies. The most common reason for the delayed payments was simply that the carriers purported they had never received the claims that we had sent.

Insurance company tactics for delaying payments include the following:

1. Simply not responding to claims. The most common tactic employed by insurance companies is simply not to respond to submitted claims. A medical practice must have an efficient way to make sure that claims are sent, received by the insurance carriers, and followed through to payment. Although it is the responsibility of the insurance companies to process all claims, it is not their responsibility to make sure that all claims are received. Because of the obvious difficulty in proving that an insurer's system has not received a claim, the insurer can easily say, "we never received your claim" as a reason for not paying, even in cases where medical practices have received electronic confirmation of receipt. This is common. No matter how sophisticated one's billing software may be, insurance carriers can still deny the receipt of claims, and there is not much the practice can do about it. One can easily speculate that insurance carriers are simply hoping that physicians do not follow up on unacknowledged claims, so the insurance will never have to pay.

2. Asking questions or asking for chart notes. If a claim is injury related, the insurance carriers will often ask for chart notes and contact the patient, because they want to ask about the nature of the injury. This is to make sure the injury is not an auto accident or work related, for which they can legally deny the claim. If the patient does not respond, the claim can simply become lost in their system until a practice's billing team detects the nonpayment.

3. Playing games with bill modifiers. A modifier is a number that is attached to a procedure code upon billing the insurer so that it prompts the insurer to pay for the procedure in addition to the office visit code. If a modifier is not attached to the code, the code will not be paid and this nonpayment can go undetected if the practice does not have a good way to screen for them. Insurance carriers generally do not seek to remedy the omission of a modifier code, even when it is obvious.

Certain procedures are commonly billed with modifiers while others are not. Forgetting to attach a modifier will result in a nonpayment. However, other codes that normally do not require a modifier can also be unexpectedly denied payment at any time. My practice has encountered such sudden, unexpected denial of payments for procedures that were paid in the past without use of a modifier in the billing code. The discovery of the nonpayments only came about because I started performing random audits. Other practices could easily be cheated of the payments they deserve if insurers decided not to pay claims for myriad reasons, such as suddenly requiring a modifier on normally paid procedures without informing the medical practice.

For example, during the first half of the 2000s, procedures such as injections or nebulizer breathing treatments were paid, along with each office visit, by health plans without any problem and without a modifier. Then one day I started noticing that the payment for each of the two procedures had stopped. The first nonpayment by this particular health plan was not detected until several months down the road when I performed a random audit and came across the nonpayment for the nebulizer breathing treatment that had always been paid by the health plan in the past. The representative for the health plan did not know why the denial occurred and admitted that it should have been paid. Upon further questioning, the health plan administrator stated that a "modifier" to the coding was supposed to be used when billing the procedure. A modifier historically was not required for simple procedures such as rapid strep test, urinalysis, taking x-rays, starting an IV, and giving nebulizer treatments, and so forth. Failure of the insurance provider to inform my practice of these changes would have net them thousands of dollars over time had I not been vigilant. How many medical practices failed to catch on, I wonder.

Since the first occurrence, there have been similar denials by other insurance plans as well. The point here is that doctors and their practices may not even know or detect these denials because no notice is given, allowing insurance companies to keep the money longer and maybe permanently.

4. Denying certain diagnoses automatically. Doctor visits can be denied payment if the visits are for certain diagnoses, even if these diagnoses present as serious medical problems. Examples of such diagnoses are: obesity, tobacco abuse, alcohol abuse, and temporomandibular joint disorder (TMJ), among others. Many doctors, including myself, are frustrated with the denial of payment for these diagnoses because such problems are real and require medical attention. Health insurance companies simply will not cover these problems, presumably because they believe coverage of such lifestyle-dependent diseases can further promote the very lifestyles that are disease promoting.

5. Threatening to audit and downcoding. A few years ago, an executive of a health insurance company called and asked to meet with me. He sent a certified letter before the call stating that his company's analysis of the claims that our practice had sent in the prior year showed too many level-IV office visits when compared to level-III. (A level-IV office visit is one in which the severity and complexity of the illness or injury warrants more time; these are reimbursed about $30 to $40 more than an office visit level-III.) He stated that this excess was outside of the norm when compared to other doctors in the same area. He also requested that our medical records be audited to ensure our compliance with coding regulations. I replied that since we are walk-in, urgent care clinics, it logically followed that the severity and complexity of the visits would be higher than regular checkups performed by family doctors, therefore occasioning frequent higher levels of office visit.

After the audit, I never heard from him again. My point for discussing such a tactic of auditing is that many doctors around the country are scared of being audited by insurance companies. It can create anxiety for the doctors because the contract to see the members for that particular health plan can be threatened. Many of my own physician employees and other physicians nationwide end up "downcoding" their visit claims to stay under the radar in order to avoid confrontation with health insurance auditors and risk losing their contracts. After my encounter with the insurance executive, I was left wondering if his letter was intended to urge me into downcode the office visits to his advantage.

According to David Doyle, CEO CRT Medical Systems, one of the top 100 largest medical billing companies, many physicians tend to be cautious with their coding and use a lower billing code instead of billing at appropriate levels out of fear of an audit. *Medical Economics* estimates that physicians who routinely downcode lose an estimated $40,000 to $50,000 in annual revenue.

6. Denying payment for legitimate codes. Urgent care clinics, including mine, are open late into the evenings, on weekends, and on holidays. There are several codes that we can use to bill in addition to an office visit in order to be reimbursed for the extra expense of offering extended clinic hours. Additionally, some urgent care clinics employ registered nurses and radiology technicians—who cost more to employ—to perform specialized procedures that are not normally performed in regular family doctor clinics, such as IVs and x-rays. These extra expenses help prevent patients from going to emergency rooms, saving both patients and their insurance carriers from higher medical costs.

I've had face-to-face talks with major health insurance company representatives who acknowledged the extra savings and the financial importance of urgent care clinics and after-hours clinics in preventing their members from going to ERs and hospitals. They even thanked me for our help in this regard. Nonetheless, when some of these insurance carriers are asked to reimburse us for these special codes to help out with our increased costs of operation, most of them say no. In the early 2000s insurance companies would pay for some of these codes, but later discontinued payment. The reason they gave is, "We follow Medicare rules and have stopped paying for these codes because Medicare does not pay for them." These are Medicare-approved codes, but even Medicare would not reimburse for them, end of story.

Here are some of the codes that have been denied payment, while urgent care and after-hours clinics continue to shoulder the increased cost of operation for the services they provide:

- 99051 – services provided in the office during regularly scheduled evening, weekend, or holiday office hours, in addition to basic service
- 99058 – services provided on an emergency basis in addition to basic service
- 99053 – services provided between 10 p.m. and 8 a.m. at 24-hour facility
- S9088 – services provided in an urgent care center

Negative Impact on Physician Practices

So far it is clear that insurance carriers employ various tactics (though legally allowed) that negatively impact the health and finances of consumers and the well-being of medical practices.

As pointed out earlier, medical practices, especially those of basic care providers, are having a difficult time maintaining their operations because nonpayment, delayed payment, and excessive investment of time, money, and energy necessary to get paid. The biggest reason, however, is the decrease in patient volume. The revenue of a medical clinic always starts with the number of patients that come into the clinic each day. We already established that doctors are required to see ever-increasing numbers of patients just to make ends meet. If there are not enough patients, then there is not enough revenue to sustain that clinic financially. Clinics are struggling nationwide because there are fewer patients going to see their doctors. This decrease is due to higher copays and higher deductibles from insurance company cost-shifting to patients.

Patient Balances Difficult to Collect

In addition to doctor practices having fewer patient visits due to higher copays, insurance company cost-shifting to insured individuals is making the collection of patient balances even more difficult for medical practices. To begin with, outstanding balances are higher these days.

Most, if not all, medical practices will agree that collecting balances from patients is much harder than from insurance companies, with less success overall. After claim processing, if a patient has a deductible that has not been met, insurance sends back an EOB (Explanation Of Benefit) about a month later, stating that the contractual payment for the entire patient visit is the patient's responsibility. An invoice is then generated by the practice and sent to the patient. Most patients will pay, but some either will not or cannot. My practice's statistics, as mentioned before, show that 70% of these patient balances will be paid three to six months after the visit and the rest (30%) will be sent to collection for more than 120 days delinquency. In other words, the $100 for a visit that used to be paid one to two months later is now paid at 70% to 80% of its full value three to six months later.

One might be tempted to argue that unpaid balances owed by patients are not the fault of insurance companies. This may be true because the patients choose these higher deductible plans. Nonetheless, in theory, these patients should not have to pay for their medical expenses at all because they have "insurance," thus defeating the very purpose it purports to serve. This contradiction is now prompting us to look into the true cause of our healthcare problems, which will be discussed in detail in Chapter 5.

Using Health to Make Money

I had a chance to go on a medical mission to Haiti in October 2012 and 2013. We were providing basic medical care out of a school in a small town with a population of seven thousand with no running water or electricity. This "temporary" clinic is made available to this town twice a year by a non-profit organization called My Aid to Haiti. For the rest of the year, the residents have no medical facility. The closest medical clinic is a 45-minute drive away, but since townspeople have no means of transportation to that clinic they continue to live their lives with bladder infections, heartburn, stomach ulcers, back pain, and even broken bones while waiting for the biannual clinic to open its doors.

What I learned from these mission is that we have abundant medical resources in the United States but we are not using them for the right purposes. Our medical assets are being used to generate income. Residents of a country like Haiti would love to have even a fraction of what we have in order to take care of even the most basic needs, such as antibiotics for bladder infections, Tylenol® for back pain, and Maalox® for stomach pain. Despite our abundant medical resources, there are still millions of Americans who are not able to access proper care. They might as well be living in a town with medical services for only a few weeks each year, as do my patients in Haiti.

It should be obvious at this point that our healthcare industry is all about making money. Our health and its needs are being used to create excessive, expensive medical procedures and treatment modalities with the primary focus of generating revenue. This focus on revenue increases the medical care costs for everyone in this country, thus compromising the health of everyone. Medical conglomerates, insurance companies, and other for-profit (and nonprofit) entities in our healthcare industry generate billions of dollars in revenue while many argue that it's good for the economy and is an inevitable byproduct of our free enterprise system.

There is no such thing as billions and billions of dollars being transacted through the healthcare sector in countries like Haiti because there the objective is to meet the basic medical needs of the general public. Such a system does not have high costs, does not have high insurance premiums, and does not force people into bankruptcy due to medical balances because the true purpose of its healthcare system, the little that they have, is to meet needs, as opposed to making money as in our current system. Such a system as that found in Haiti, which is on the opposite end of the spectrum to that of US healthcare, is not what we want. Nevertheless, a happy medium—the solution—must be somewhere in between. The bottom line is that a healthcare system should be created and maintained for the right reason—to provide needed medical care, not to generate excessive corporate profits.

Five

Chapter 5
The Root Cause

I began this book with a discussion of how the US population started shifting to the use of emergency rooms in the 1950s and how this worsened to the point where the traditional model of receiving care from independent family doctors transformed into one-stop healthcare shopping mall provided by conglomerates, resulting in a drastic increase in healthcare costs. Then I discussed how health insurance companies contribute to the problem, driving costs higher while using various tactics on both patients and medical practices in order to increase revenue and profit.

From this discussion, one may think that I am pointing my finger at our ERs, hospitals, healthcare conglomerates, and health insurance companies for breaking our private healthcare system. I am not.

I have simply pointed out what has been taking place over the last several years. This chapter will demonstrate that healthcare conglomerates and private health insurance companies are not, in and of themselves, the causes of the crisis of our private healthcare system. I will point to the root cause of our healthcare problems—the system itself and the under-regulated dynamic between entities within the system.

Again, please keep in mind that this book is discussing only the private sector of our healthcare system and not directly referring to any government-sponsored program such as Medicare, Medicaid, or the VA system, their problems or potential solutions. The government sector is a complicated system. It requires a deeper understanding and more complicated solution, which is a the subject for another book.

Are Healthcare Providers the Cause?

It may seem from Chapter 3 that one main cause of our healthcare problems are healthcare providers—the doctors, clinics, emergency rooms, hospitals, and healthcare conglomerates who regularly perform more tests and treatments than necessary and bill exorbitant rates for them. But they are not the root cause of our healthcare problems. They are a necessary part of the solution.

The rising costs of medical care, as concerns practitioners, stem from the fee-for-service method that our system has allowed to go on without limit—that is, the more services provided, the more fees charged, and the greater the profit. Healthcare providers do what they have to do in order to survive, and hopefully make a profit as business entities. They will push our current system to the limit and get paid even if they order procedures for no good reason—to avoid lawsuits, to make profit, or simply because they don't know what they are doing.

In other words, the root cause of the increasing medical care costs is simply the system itself—the dynamic between healthcare providers and insurance companies who both have a profit motive and attempt to manipulate earnings by adapting to each others' cost-saving and cost-making ploys.

Are Health Insurance Companies the Cause?

It may also be apparent from Chapter 4 that another main cause of our broken healthcare system are health insurance companies that want to maximize profits using whatever means they can. They have been increasing their premiums significantly each year for the last several years.

In February 2010, the *Los Angeles Times* reported that Anthem Blue Cross of California announced multiple rate increases across the state, averaging 30% to 35% for hundreds of thousands of its members, causing uproar among the public, the media, and politicians including President Obama. The outrage led Anthem to settle for lower rate increases. I can see why so many people were upset with Anthem for such actions and why they accused it of being unreasonable and caring about nothing but profits. Nonetheless, the public did not see the real reason behind the push for such rate increases or the federal and state regulations that health insurance companies must follow.

Not many people know that health insurance companies have to turn in their health plans' designs and prices to the government annually, by the end of April, nine months before they can start selling the plans the following January. This means that they would not have all of the annual data from these plans' usage in the first year for analysis to make any necessary adjustments before they have to turn the designs and prices into the government again for the next year. This also means that if they design their plans and price them incorrectly, they could operate at a loss for two years before they have sufficient usage data to adjust their plan designs and prices to bring them out of the negative. So in 2010 and 2011, without knowing what the upcoming impact of Obamacare was going to be, health insurance companies sought to maximize profit as much as they could while they could, and premiums rose significantly. Would it be fair then to blame health insurance companies exclusively for such bothersome rate increases each year? I think not. It is in part the system that prompted them to behave this way.

Just like healthcare providers and healthcare conglomerates, our health insurance companies are not, in and of themselves, the root cause of our healthcare problems. Health insurance is a necessary part of our lives just like doctors, clinics, and hospitals.

Health insurance premiums keep rising for three reasons:

1. Fee-for-service billing allows medical providers to overcharge and overprescribe unnecessary procedures.
2. The McCarran-Ferguson Act limits competition among health

insurance companies resulting in collusion and a lack of competitive premium pricing.

3. For decades consumers have received medical care and procedures without knowing the price because "my insurance covers everything."

Just like healthcare providers, health insurance companies will continue to do what they can do, and have to do, in order to make as much profit as possible. In other words, the root cause of rising health insurance premiums is the system itself and the fee-for-service dynamic between healthcare providers and insurance companies that continues without any sort of capitation or intervention.

A perfect example to demonstrate this interplay, and the allowance by the system for cost escalation, is a medical situation encountered by one of my editors, Katy. Katy's car was rear-ended one day by a truck. The impact jammed her right leg against her hip, painfully misaligning the sacroiliac (SI) joint of her pelvis and lower back. She was evaluated by an osteopathic doctor, who subsequently and performed manipulative therapy during many visits, but without improvement, in his private osteopathic office. After seeing the same doctor often and without improvement, Katy finally asked him why he kept asking her to make appointments for her unresolved pain. The doctor responded, "It is necessary in order to make your case appear significant so the insurance company will cover your claims." She felt distrustful of this doctor and sought the help of a well-known physical therapist who finally resolved her SI joint pain after a few sessions. She paid cash for this therapist, but the amount was far less than what the car insurer paid the osteopathic doctor.

In conclusion, it was not necessarily the doctor who escalated the cost of Katy's care, but the interplay between him and the insurance company encouraged by our fee-for-service system. Once Katy bypassed this system and paid cash, she resolved her problem at far less cost. Significantly, Katy's medical problem would not have otherwise been resolved.

Since insurance companies receive wasteful claims from cases like Katy's, they have naturally developed tactics to handle such abuse, minimize their payout, and maximize their revenue. Likewise doctors, in order to receive adequate reimbursement from insurance carriers, continue to prescribe unnecessary office visits and procedures to keep their practices afloat.

Health insurance companies are an important part of our lives. We need them to remain in this private insurance market and help us, just like we need our healthcare providers. We just need the two forces to work together in a new way—the dynamic between the two needs to change.

The Root Cause

As we go through our daily lives, we all find ourselves caught up in systems or situations that force us to do certain things if we want to survive. The same is true for healthcare providers and health insurance companies. They are in it to operate successful businesses and to make profits.

The system and the dynamic that has developed among its agents over the decades is the root cause of our healthcare crisis. Our healthcare system has evolved into something that is not balanced, as illustrated by the following two diagrams. Figure 1 (next page) shows a balanced dynamic among consumers, providers, and insurance carriers where all three entities have enough cash on hand which allows them to exert equal control on the healthcare system. In this balanced dynamic, the premium is not too expensive, enabling consumers to keep some cash in their pockets while giving enough cash to the insurance carriers for them to pay medical claims (1) and enjoy a modest profit. The copay and deductibles are low enough not to deter consumers from visiting doctors and hospitals (2, 3, and 4), allowing providers to earn enough revenue to keep their businesses going (5 and 6). This was our healthcare system of yesterday which is now being thrown off balance.

Figure 2, on the following page, shows our current imbalanced healthcare system. Consumers are paying high premiums for their health insurance (1), along with higher copays and deductibles (2). The higher copays and deductibles result in fewer visits to doctors and hospitals, which leads to two things: serious illness that requires costlier services, and efforts by doctors and hospitals to compensate for lost revenue (3). Economic pressures and the need to generate more revenue and profits motivate doctors, medical

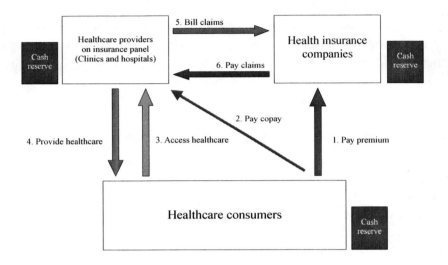

Figure 1. The balanced healthcare dynamic

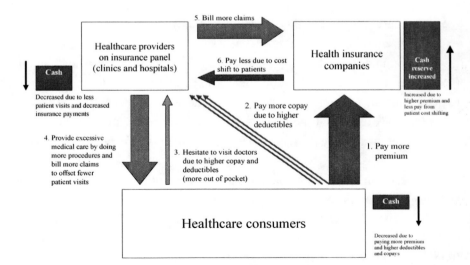

Figure 2. The imbalanced healthcare dynamic

practices, and healthcare conglomerates to perform more procedures (4). Overutilization substantially increases claims to health insurance companies (5). More claims inflate health insurance premiums, causing more shifting of cash into health insurers' pockets. Medical practices want to get more of this cash, so they do more procedures and bill more claims.

The cycle repeats in a snowball effect that further tilts the imbalance in the private healthcare sector. It is not a healthy dynamic but a system heading for disaster.

Our system is heading in the wrong direction and is negatively affecting people's health and finances. It is negatively impacting the growth of small businesses and their ability to take care of their employees. While most employers are still able to provide health insurance plans despite the increasing premiums, other employers are finding ways to avoid the requirement to provide these benefits. One way is limiting their business growth by keeping the number of full-time employees to fewer than than 50. Another way is to limit employees' work week to 29 hours or less, as Utah's Granite School district threatened its 5,200 hourly employees (as reported by Tom Wharton of the *Salt Lake Tribune* on May 2, 2013).

Since there is no way to cap health insurance premiums, they may continue to grow until enough employers will choose to pay penalties rather than offer employee health benefits that insurance pools will become unable to pay medical claims. One large nutritional company in Salt Lake City has already voiced a plan to not provide insurance and pay the penalties because they're less expensive. In the end, health insurers will have to exit the market, forcing our government to step in and provide centralized healthcare—the ultimate demise of our private healthcare system that few of us want to see.

In order to formulate a solution, we need to understand how our systemic dysfunction began and became what it is.

How Health Insurance Was Born

Health insurance is basically a prepaid health membership system. While accident insurance has existed since the 1850s, our current system began in the late 1920s when Dr. Michael Shadid in Elk City, Oklahoma accepted a fixed monthly fee in exchange for his medical services. The prepaid model, the precursor to our current health insurance industry, was born. The prepaid model quickly extended to include hospital care because the innovative concept gained interest and was adopted by multiple clinics and hospitals. For example, in 1929 Ross-Loos Medical Group became one of the first and largest prepaid systems. It included 29 clinics and 1 multi-specialty hospital in the Los Angeles area. In 1982 the group eventually transformed into Cigna, the health insurance giant of today. A similar program was created in 1945 by industrialist Henry Kaiser and later became Kaiser Permanente health system, one of the largest HMOs in the nation.

Around the same time that Dr. Shadid started his prepayment program in the 1920s, a group of 1,500 schoolteachers in Dallas approached Baylor University Hospital and negotiated three weeks prepaid care for a fixed payment of $6 per person per year. Justin Ford Kimball, an official for Baylor University, accepted the prepaid plan, paving the way for the creation of Blue Cross health plans.

The Transformation

The practice of prepaying for medical care initially involved prepayment directly to doctors and the hospitals for whatever limited services they could provide. Then it quickly transformed to prepaying a third-party administrator—a middleman—instead. This allowed members to access larger health systems and more facilities. This is the birth of the US health insurance industry—Blue Cross being the first insurance company. (Blue Shield was founded a few years later.)

The beauty of these health insurance plans was that they increasingly allowed members to access a variety of medical procedures at a variety of hospitals and doctors across the country, as opposed to limited procedures by fewer doctors and hospitals in a given geographical area. This is when consumers started to pay higher prices for their medical care—when control of the healthcare dollar shifted from the hands of consumers and medical providers to the hands of health insurance companies. This shift in financial control was subtle and happened early enough so that recent generations have become accustomed to it, thinking that it is the norm and even inevitable. No one ever thought at the time that so simple a shift would later result in the significant hardships that doctors and consumers now endure.

For several decades after its beginning in the 1920s, health insurance premiums, although slowly rising, were for the most part financially tolerable and affordable by consumers and their employers. One reason the premiums remained tolerable was there were many smaller health insurance companies throughout the nation, amidst the giants like Blue Cross Blue Shield, UnitedHealthcare, and Cigna, competing with one another for customers. Such competition helped keep the premiums down.

Then the market underwent drastic change. According to a Zacks Equity Research report published in 2012, since 1996 the healthcare industry witnessed acquisitions worth approximately $90 billion, resulting in dominance by a few players. From 1990 to 2000 there were approximately four hundred big and small mergers and acquisitions, decreasing the competition among insurance companies. The McCarran-Ferguson Act of 1945 made the situation worse, resulting in the eventual collapse of competition in the health insurance market.

Currently the market is dominated by fewer than ten health insurance giants who are often accused of collusion and price fixing. In 2010 the American Medical Association reported that the two largest insurers had a combined market share of 70% or more in 24 out of 43 states in its study. This was an increase from the prior year when 18 out of 42 states had two insurers with a combined market share of 70% or more. Also, 120 million Americans (of approximately 150 millions who are privately insured) currently receive health coverage from only seven large publicly traded health insurance companies. (See *Competition in Health Insurance: A Comprehensive Study of U.S. Markets.*)

Larger and stronger health insurance companies mean less control by members. Instead of prepaying a few dollars to a doctor or a hospital for whatever limited medical services we needed to maintain our health, we began to pay more, and to the middlemen. In exchange, we received fancier and more complicated health plans with access to every kind of medical procedure and treatment from a variety of healthcare providers across the country. Now taken to the extreme, we pay top dollar for these fancy health membership plans with special features we rarely use. We typically only go to one doctor, one clinic, or one hospital (if we ever need hospitalization). It is like paying for a Cadillac that we never drive—it sits in the garage while we ride a bike to the store down the street for all our basic needs.

To summarize, the shift from prepaying healthcare providers directly to prepaying the middleman has resulted in loss of control of healthcare dollars by consumers and medical providers.

Putting It Simply

In conclusion, the healthcare system itself is the root cause of our healthcare crisis because it fosters a dysfunctional dynamic. The fee-for-service system has escalated the price of medical services, especially when compared to the actual cost of providing those services. The system enables middlemen to control the private healthcare sector, charging high premiums as they try to recover the costs of overused advanced medical care and pay a substantial returns to their shareholders. In the meantime, consumers agreed to access services without giving thought to price because they have good employers who provided good insurance that conveniently "covered everything."

Our system now fails us: It causes financial stress, higher mortality rates, and less access to needed medical care. We simply need to rationalize medical care costs by avoiding the unnecessary use of advanced medicine and begin to regulate reimbursements for procedures ordered outside medical guidelines. We also need to use health insurance middleman more appropriately for costs we absolutely cannot afford while taking direct care of costs we can afford.

Six

Chapter 6
The Solution

The final objective of this book is to suggest action that we can take to work in conjunction with the new healthcare law and the many changes it brings. Obamacare is here to stay and our healthcare system is undergoing the biggest change in its history, one that will effect us all one way or another.

Unfortunately because Obamacare alone will not fix the three major problems we have discussed, our private healthcare system is headed for a cliff sooner rather than later. The good news is that we can do something about it. The time is right to create a revolution and change our healthcare system for the better.

The rest of this book will explore how we can take advantage of Obamacare to contain and reduce healthcare costs; use health insurance more appropriately and affordably; and enable our family doctors, their practices, and even health conglomerates to meet our essential health care needs more effectively.

Obamacare: a Brief Overview

Before I proceed in detail on how we can work together to create our healthcare revolution, I believe it is important for all of us to have a bird's eye view of Obamacare. The American Public Health Association has put together a nice summary of the Affordable Care Act (ACA) for us:

Obamacare has two major areas of reforms: insurance reform and health system reform.

A. Insurance Reform

a. The law helps increase health coverage by: 1) allowing young adults to stay on their parents' plans until the age of 26; 2) expanding Medicaid coverage by lowering eligibility; 3) banning denial of coverage by insurers due to preexisting conditions; 4) allowing individuals to shop for competitive coverage online via an "Insurance Exchange"; 5) mandating individuals to purchase health plans or pay a fine; and 6) mandating employers with 50 or more full-time employees to provide health insurance with a maximum level of employee contribution.

b. The law also increases insurance benefits by: 1) requiring insurers to cover certain preventive services without extra costs to members; and 2) requiring insurers to provide a minimum set of benefits in order to participate in the Insurance Exchange.

c. The law protects consumers by: 1) prohibiting insurers from charging high premiums based on health status or gender; 2) banning coverage limits on certain essential benefits; and 3) requiring insurers to make their coverage and benefits clear to consumers so consumers can easily make comparisons with other health plans.

d. The law lowers costs for consumers by: 1) forcing insurers to make profit and administrative costs fit within 20% of their premium income (15% of premiums from groups of 100 or more employees), otherwise the excess must be refunded to their members; 2) providing subsidies to many small businesses for buying exchange plans; and 3) requiring insurers to justify, on the state level, any annual premium increases of 10% or more.

B. Health System Reform

a. The law improves quality of care and efficiency by: 1) giving Medicare incentives to providers who coordinate to improve quality of care via Accountable Care Organizations; 2) promoting medical home models of coordinating care and integrating medical services; 3) implementing new quality measures for various care parameters and outcomes; and 4) limiting Medicare payments based on quality measurements.

    b. The law attempts to make the workforce stronger by: 1) increasing Medicaid payments to equal Medicare payments; 2) increasing funding to community health centers and school-based health centers; 3) increasing Medicare primary care payment by a 10% bonus; 4) increasing funding for providers who serve communities in need; and 5) increasing funding for training in public health and preventive medicine.

    c. The law finally emphasizes greater focus on public health and prevention by increasing funding in various programs such as: the Prevention & Public Health Fund (PPHF), Community Transformation Grants (CTG), and Community Health Needs Assessments (CHNAs).

As we can see, this overview does not convey a full understanding of the law but that's not necessary for the purposes of this book. The actual Affordable Healthcare Act contains more than 20,000 pages and stands over seven feet tall when printed out, making it one of the most complicated laws in history.

Throughout this book I refer to the ACA as "Obamacare" because I truly believe President Obama deserves the credit for what he and his administration have done. This health reform law may be controversial to some, wholly unacceptable to many, and disliked by others, but it offers two pieces that are especially significant to our discussion.

The first piece is the famous Obamacare insurance mandate, and it's complicated. But in general, individuals who are capable of paying income taxes and who are not eligible for Medicaid or Medicare must purchase a health insurance plan for themselves and their dependents or else face an annual tax penalty. Also, employers with more than 50 full-time employees must provide health insurance coverage for full-time employees or else face a hefty annual penalty.

The second significant piece is the limitation that Obamacare places on the profit margins of health insurance companies. The mandate states that 80% of premiums from small employee groups and 85% of premiums from larger employee groups (100 or more) must be used to pay medical claims, leaving only 20% and 15%, respectively, for health insurance companies to cover their administrative costs and profits. These two pieces play a significant role in the solution we can create together.

Obamacare: Paving the Way

Mandating enrollment and capping profits appear brilliant to Obamacare supporters, but a deeper look reveals flaws. Although an increase in insurance funds will cover medical expenses for more insured people, and the funds cannot be taken excessively by health insurance companies via profits, the funds can still become dangerously depleted.

Funds will be depleted when: 1) medical practices, ERs, hospitals, and healthcare conglomerates perform unnecessary procedures for purposes of making profit; and 2) insurers continue to pay for certain medical care that should not be paid for by insurance funds and that can be affordably taken care of by consumers themselves.

While Obamacare alone will break down when insurance funds are depleted, we—consumers and medical providers—can help preserve insurance funds for use on more appropriate and costly expenses, while taking care of our basic medical care ourselves in various innovative ways.

Otherwise, if we do not step in together to take action and help make Obamacare work, the three main problems that we are currently having, described in the first half of this book, will worsen: medical care costs will keep on rising; insurance premiums will proportionally escalate; and we will have fewer family doctors and more healthcare conglomerates geared toward profit—a snowball effect that will likely pick up speed as the mandate takes effect for individuals in January 2014 and for employers in January of 2015.

The transformation of our private healthcare system over the recent years, prior to Obamacare, was driven by this healthcare snowball effect and has led us to intervention by our government and an increase in governmental control over our private healthcare system. It has led us to a point where if we move forward without a supplement to Obamacare, the snowball effect will get worse, prompting more governmental control down the road if we do not step in and help prevent it now.

The Two Missing Keys

What's missing from Obamacare? Obamacare paves way for healthcare improvement by requiring more insurance funds to be made available to cover more claims for more people. It also protects these funds from being depleted by excess profit taking. This results in a bigger chunk of funds available to cover healthcare costs for everyone...theoretically. In practice if those funds are intended to cover both basic and advanced care, and usage remains uncontrolled, then the funds cannot cover everyone's healthcare expenses.

Because Obamacare lacks the first key—control of medical care expenses—it will not reduce health insurance premiums as President Obama promised.

The first key is the most important, and without it Obamacare will fail to repair our healthcare crisis. Medical care costs in this country will continue to increase as long as: 1) there is no legal or effective regulation on the ordering of unnecessary procedures or the pricing of those procedures; and 2) there is no incentive for medical practices to discontinue ordering excess procedures or keep their costs down for patients other than those who use Medicare and Medicaid. This will erode insurance funds continuously, causing health insurers to raise premiums.

Obamacare supporters may argue that Accountable Care Organizations (ACOs)—a provision of the new law which gives bonuses and incentives to doctors for improving outcomes while keeping the costs down—will address the need for cost control. However, this incentive will not work in controlling the overall costs because it only pays for care given to Medicare and Medicaid patients, and not privately insured patients (as of this printing). Additionally, the law does not impose any legal restrictions on ordering and being paid for unnecessary procedures or on using the RVU system in paying doctors' salaries—both of which are major causes of rising costs.

A "reasonable standard of care" in medical practice has been set for most, if not all, illnesses and conditions by our training and academic institutions. This reasonable standard of care has been developed over decades and adapted to changing technology, yet it is not used these days to promote cost control in our healthcare system. It is used, however, to control costs in healthcare systems in other countries around the world. To create the first missing key to Obamacare, and in order to start controlling overall healthcare costs, someone must step in and effectively implement a reasonable standard of care. It may as well be us—providers and consumers—who step in do this before our government does. The rest of this book will discuss how we can take such action.

The second missing key is the lack of competition among health insurance companies that are being protected from federal antitrust laws by the The McCarran-Ferguson Act. Obamacare supporters may argue that the profit margin limitation on health insurance companies will normalize the profits that health insurance companies can make across the board and bring premium prices down. I would argue that this is not the same as allowing full-blown, naturally occurring competition to take place, in which case there would be many more competitors in the insurance market (rather than the current "Big 10") who could potentially bring premium prices down even more than what results from the Obamacare profit margin limitation. This cannot take place as long as the The McCarran-Ferguson Act is still in place.

While the Obamacare Insurance Exchange are designed to promote competition among existing health insurance companies, and may promote the creation of new insurance companies, it cannot guarantee it as long as the The McCarran-Ferguson Act remains in place. Moreover, new grounds for competition among healthcare providers and their own health plans are additionally needed to bring health insurance premiums down. This is the subject of the next chapter.

Until the two missing keys are addressed, health insurance premiums will rise continuously. If the first key is in place, limiting usage to a reasonable standard of care, then medical care costs will come down along with premiums. If the second key is in place, the restoration of antitrust regulation, then the health insurance profit margin might dip below the allowed 15% to 20% and lower premiums altogether.

How We Can Help Fix Our Healthcare

Controlling medical care costs and bringing down insurance premiums are the two essential tasks left to us in order to save our private healthcare system. No one else can effectively accomplish these tasks but we, consumers and practitioners, because no one else truly has our best interests at heart. Only we can effectively make this happen. We are the only ones that have the ability to effectively shift billions of dollars back into our own pockets and bank accounts. Such a shift will open the door to competition, not just among health insurers but also among healthcare providers, including conglomerates. Most of all, this shift will help preserve insurance funds, reserving them for more expensive and necessary medical procedures and preventing insurance premiums from rising.

In order to understand how we can help achieve these two goals, we must understand one basic concept—expected care versus unexpected loss. It is the understanding of this basic concept that will allow us to become more strategic about how we approach our own healthcare and spend our healthcare dollars, thus resulting in cost control and encouraging competition.

Expected Care versus Unexpected Loss

There is a good reason why the auto insurance industry does not have skyrocketing premiums. While it would be nice if oil changes and car engine repairs were paid by our auto insurance, we would be paying sky-high auto premiums like that of our health insurance. Our auto insurance premium remains low because it only pays for unexpected losses such as collisions. So why does health insurance pay for everything from expected, regular checkups to unexpected organ transplants?

First, we must divide healthcare providers into two categories of services as discussed in Chapter 2: basic care and advanced care. Basic care services meet *expected* needs and include annual checkups, maintenance of chronic problems, as well as caring for minor illnesses and injuries that one may expect as a normal part of life. Advanced care services include care given as a result of *unexpected* events that are costly and can be catastrophic such as major accidents, cancer, stroke, or heart attack. Health insurance has been paying for both expected and unexpected expenses since the 1920s.

Imagine this comparison as the single biggest difference between car insurance and health insurance. Let's compare the total cost of an oil change for all insured cars in the nation to the total cost of repairing all cars involved in accidents. According to the U.S. Bureau of Transportation Statistics, in 2009 there were 254,212,610 registered vehicles in the United States. Of this number, there were estimated to have been 5,505,000 auto accidents, which is one crash in 46 million cars. The per capita cost for car crashes varies from $600 to $1,200 for each state with the nationwide average being $819, according to the Rocky Mountain Insurance Information Association. This means that the cost of repairing the 5,505,000 crashes is approximately 4.5 billion dollars. In contrast, if an oil change costs $50 per car, the total cost of doing oil changes for all 254,212,610 registered cars would be 12.7 billion dollars per oil change. Twice a year oil change would cost 25.4 billion dollars and four times a year would cost 50.8 billion dollars. Either cost dwarfs our 4.5 billion in accident repairs.

Furthermore, if your auto mechanic knew that your auto insurance would pay for changing oil, fluids, brake pads, engine repair, and everything else that is elective, they would probably not hesitate to do as much repair work as possible and perform maintenance as frequently as possible. You would probably not hesitate to allow this upon their recommendation, *and knowing that your insurance would cover it.*

In parallel with our auto insurance scenario, let's compare the cost of doing surgery for appendicitis to the cost of giving all insured people a checkup. Our incidence of appendicitis is 1 in 400 or 0.25%, which equals 788,932 appendicitis surgeries in our current population of 315,573,000. According to the Healthcare Blue Book, an appendectomy costs $13,351 on average. This puts a total cost of appendectomies for our US population at $10.5 billion. On the other hand, there are approximately 196 million Americans with private health insurance in the United States. If each insured receives a checkup for $100 per visit, then the total cost is $19.6 billion, and four doctor's visits per year (the average in the United States) comes to $78.4 billion.

Note that $78.4 billion in checkups and regular doctor visits, our *expected* expenses, dwarf our *unexpected* expense of $10.5 billion for appendectomies in collective terms.

Now imagine the health insurance premium designed to cover costs of checkups and appendectomies versus the premium for appendectomies alone. There's little wonder that the United States is the biggest spender of healthcare in the world and that our insurance premiums are prohibitively high.

The takeaway from this comparison between health insurance and car insurance is that covering the expenses for expected, basic care services is what is causing our health insurance premiums to be so high. In other words, it is the main predator that depletes the pool of insurance funds more effectively than anything else, including profits taken by health insurance companies. This is why Obamacare by itself cannot resolve our health affordability crisis and why US medical care costs and health insurance premiums will keep rising with no end in sight.

Our first solution, therefore, is to begin paying for our own basic medical care and expected services if we want to have lower insurance premiums. This is essential to achieving our first missing key—medical cost control.

Stay Healthy at a Fixed Cost—the Capitation Model

If you have no idea how much mechanics in your area would charge you for an oil change for your car, wouldn't you likely hesitate to get an oil change? This situation is just like not knowing how much you will owe a clinic before seeing your doctor, only to be surprised after your insurance is billed. On the other hand, if local mechanics have set prices, only differing slightly from one another, you can price shop and make the oil change fit your budget. You are now in control of your oil changes because the cost is known and controlled by competition. Wouldn't it be nice if visiting a doctor worked the same way—knowing the total cost of care and knowing it will be low due to competition? Currently there is no price competition among medical practices because the prices for care are not known at the time of service and are determined by each patient's health insurance plan after the claims are processed. One can imagine the impossibility of budgeting and price control by consumers and providers when it comes to healthcare.

Further, the cost can escalate without your knowledge if your health insurance is billed for the payment. This is because there are various levels of office visit, as discussed earlier, each priced on a scale that differs from one health plan to another and from one region of the country to another, even though "Medicare sets the rates." But Medicare rates also vary from one region to another, even within the same state. There's little wonder that patients feel anxious when accessing care in our current healthcare system. If we can price our oil changes, why can't we price our healthcare? Bringing price transparency into healthcare will further contribute to medical cost control. help create the first missing key.

Imagine going to your doctor and knowing beforehand which procedures will be performed and their cost. It's been done before in our healthcare history—it's called *capitation*. Capitation is defined by Wikipedia as:

> *A payment arrangement for health care service providers… It pays a physician or group of physicians a set amount for each enrolled person assigned to them, per period of time, whether or not that person seeks care. These providers generally are contracted with a type of health maintenance organization (HMO)…, which enlists the providers to care for HMO-enrolled patients. The amount of remuneration is based on the average expected health care utilization of that patient, with greater payment for patients with significant medical history. Rates are also affected by age, race, sex, type of employment, and geographical locations, as these factors typically influence the cost of providing care.*

One can imagine many reasons why such a capitation model was not popular in the past among providers just by reading the word "assigned" and analyzing the stipulations following it. Just like our current failing healthcare system, capitation did not work in the past because control was in the hands of the middleman (HMOs), not providers and patients. It shifted risk management to the providers while the payments were left up to the health insurers.

The capitation to be discussed in this chapter and book is a different kind of capitation, one controlled by healthcare providers and chosen by patients and not by middlemen or governmental agencies. This different kind of capitation has been working right under our noses for the longest time with cash clinics being the primary examples.

While most clinics and medical practices provide services under the fee-for-service model, which bills health insurance plans for payments (typically accounting for about 80% of a practice on the average), there are increasing numbers of medical practices that provide services under various kinds of fixed or capitated prices. The following are some examples of capitation models that have been utilized and that are now becoming more popular because they help consumers know exactly what they will get for exactly what price:

Cash clinics

Cash clinics were the first form of capitated healthcare delivery. As the name implies, cash clinics require payment at the time of service and have set prices for each service such as office visit, strep test, x-ray, IV hydration, etc. Examples of cash-clinic practices are Dr. Brian Forrest in Apex, North Carolina and Elmer Sisneros, PA, in Heber City, Utah. Cash clinics inform patients up front what everything will cost, the opposite of the fee-for-service method of billing health insurance that oftentimes does not know how much a patient has to pay until after hearing from the insurance provider, which can take several weeks. Unfortunately, the fee-for-service model has suppressed the popularity of cash clinics for decades.

Concierge medicine

Concierge medicine or organizations such as MDVIP based in Boca Raton, Florida, and the solo practice of Dr. Michael Jennings in Salt Lake City, Utah offer family medicine for an annual capitated fee to program members. Their fees are usually in the range of $2,000 and up per person per year. Bear in mind that not all concierge medicine practices are true capitation models. This is because some concierge practices charge annual fees for access convenience but still bill health insurance plans or the patients for the visits and the procedures performed. Such practice is similar to a typical practice that bills insurance and does not prevent cost escalation.

Workplace clinics

Workplace clinics such as OnSite Care, Inc. based in Salt Lake City, Utah is one of the pioneers in providing capitated-cost family medicine to employees of large companies, such as RC Willey Home Furnishings, a local furniture store.

Medical membership

Medical membership models provide discounted, capitated medical care for a flat monthly fee. My seven clinics in Utah, After Hours Medical, follow this model that has proven popular with individuals and families whether or not they have coverage with a regular health insurance plan. Established family medicine practices can quickly, easily, and affordably adapt to the membership model as guided by state law. Medical memberships offer the best solution to creating the first key that Obamacare is missing—medical cost control. I devote Chapter 7 to this highly successful model.

Capitation by specialists

Specialists who are willing to promote sound economic practices that work in conjunction with Obamacare have set up their practices on capitated models and will surely grow in popularity. Very soon there will be more specialists offering capitated fees for their services. Specialists who do not have a lot of procedures and who manage chronic medical problems via writing prescriptions can easily adopt this model. Other specialists with high-tech procedures, such as cataract surgery, are finding ways to offer capitated medicine. A good example is Dr. David Masihdas, OD, an ophthalmologist practicing in Salt Lake City who provides eye care at a set price of $150 a year for individuals and $400 a year for families, no matter how many visits. His members receive cataract surgery at a greatly discounted price.

Other capitation models

Other capitation models will likely evolve. Once more of us see that the capitation model eliminating middlemen and working directly with providers makes sense and is central to turning our healthcare around, the clever Americans will create and adopt even more innovative capitated models. These might eventually include hospitals, health conglomerates, and the

most advanced and most costly medical services in our country—private
cancer centers. Private and direct capitation opens a whole new frontier of
competition.

With the emergence of more cash clinics, more concierge medical practices,
more on-site workplace clinics, more medical membership clinics, and even
large programs that help connect patients to doctors for fixed, predictable
prices, there will arise competition for consumer dollars. In order to attract
business, these capitated practices might be forced to compete by increasing
quality, service levels, and by lowering their prices—whatever it takes to
give them an edge.

Receiving medical care—at least basic care—from any form of capitated
practice is a much better way for patients to save money than using a high-
deductible health plan that bills health insurance. The comparison table
below illustrates the superiority of capitation.

Let's suppose, for example, that you were to seek medical care for strep
throat, pneumonia, a laceration, and a virus in one year's time (not your best
year). Your out-of-pocket costs for the four doctor visits would look like the
following in each of three different payment scenarios: using a traditional
insurance policy, paying for services at a cash clinic, or paying for services
at a medical membership clinic.

The comparison in Table 1 above clearly shows that receiving basic
medical services from the four doctor visits costs the most when billing
health insurance, even at Medicare rates, which are the lowest in the
country (except for Medicaid). The downfall: instead of insurance paying
this $578.60 balance, the insured person has to pay this total because of
the $2,000 deductible, after having already paid $600 in premiums. The
cash clinic presents a better option of paying for these four visits from the
standpoint of out-of-pocket expense, nonetheless, the membership model
offers the best out-of-pocket savings over the long term.

The biggest advantage for using a capitation model, such as a cash clinic
or membership program, is that the prices for seeing a doctor are known
before the visit, whereas insurance billing (the fee-for-service method)
does not. The pricing in the insurance column is based on the Medicare
rate for Utah. All other private insurance plans reimburse these codes at
difference prices, varying in amount from one code to another, but always

higher than the Medicare rates. Therefore, a patient does not likely know the total cost of each visit until the claim processing is done, at which time this previously mysterious balance becomes the patient's responsibility if the annual deductible has not been met.

The costs associated with basic medical care should never be mysterious and we should pay them directly ourselves, without middlemen. We should reserve our insurance plans for covering unexpected events that, by their nature, can involve expensive procedures and long-term care.

The cost control of capitated basic care is the missing key in Obamacare. We can all step up and make Obamacare work—for our own good—in so many personal ways, while saving our healthcare system.

Cost comparison of paying for 4 doctor visits using 3 methods	Insurance ($) $2,000-Ded. Health Plan	Cash ($) 5 Minute Clinic	Membership ($) After Hours Medical
Monthly Fee	$600/family	none	$25/person
Visit 1—Strep throat			
Office visit - Level 4 (new)	159.24	65.00	10.00
Strep test	12.50	5.00	included
Visit 2—Pneumonia			
Office visit - Level 4 (established)	102.78	65.00	10.00
Chest x-ray	18.76	20.00	included
Antibiotic shot	2.88	10.00	included
IM injection	24.23	included	included
Breathing treatment	17.83	10.00	included
Visit 3—Laceration repair			
Office visit - Level 3	69.91	included	10.00
Laceration repair	88.06	110.00	included
Visit 4—Viral sore throat			
Office visit - Level 3	69.91	65.00	10.00
Strep test	12.50	5.00	included
Total out-of-pocket cost	**$578.60**	**$355.00**	**$40.00**

Table 1. Comparison of four basic care visits to a doctor's office, using three methods of payment: insurance billing ($2,000 deductible plan and reimbursed at Utah Medicare rates), paying cash at a cash clinic, and using a medical membership program such as that offered by After Hours Medical in Salt Lake City, Utah.

Cost Savings for Patients—but What about Medical Practices?

The reduction in out-of-pocket costs with the cash clinic and membership methods, as illustrated in the table below, offers a great saving for patients. A medical doctor or a health care provider looking at this comparison may quickly dismiss the membership model and wonder:

- How is it going to generate enough revenue to support a practice?
- What does this patient's savings look like in the big picture of the membership model?
- How will health insurance be utilized under the medical membership model?
- How will such a model fit in with Obamacare and its requirements?

These are great questions that the rest of this chapter and book will answer.

Let's take a look at a hypothetical example that will show how the medical membership model can be a superior way to deliver cost-saving care to patients and also generate sufficient revenue to support a medical practice. This example will demonstrate how billions of dollars in premiums can be saved and shifted to our pockets and our doctors' pockets while we ourselves control basic care costs, remain healthy, and preserve our doctor-patient relationships. At the same time insurance companies can remain viable in our free market economy—everyone wins.

Health Insurance versus Membership, a Shocking Comparison

Medical membership can reduce the cost of our basic medical needs more effectively when compared to using health insurance for the same basic needs. In other words, don't let the middleman be involved in something that you and your basic care doctors can mutually agree to take care of together at a much lower cost, much like paying for your own car oil changes and engine tune ups.

Let me demonstrate how a medical membership program can save millions of dollars in a scenario that involves taking care of a population of patients needing only basic care, while allowing the doctor and their patients to prosper financially.

Let's look at a hypothetical medical practice of a family doctor who takes care of 2,000 patients. The doctor is so good at protecting his patients' health that each visits the clinic only four times a year without any hospital admissions or any care from other facilities. (Actual statistics by a large insurance brokerage company that has been in business in Utah for a long time show that the annual number of visits to primary care doctors in Utah is 1,969 per 1,000 population. This is equivalent to twice a year per person, but I am going to use four visits a year here, as I do earlier in this book, just to be on the conservative side and because people with chronic conditions, such as diabetes or heart disease, often see their doctor up to four times per year.)

Now let's suppose two scenarios of payment: one is a traditional insurance model and the other is a membership model. In the insurance scenario, let's suppose that each patient pays $600 a month in insurance premiums to have a $500 deductible health plan. When visiting a doctor, the patient will pay a $20 copay and the insurance will pay $100 for the rest of the visit if the payment for each visit is reimbursed at $120 contractually.

In the membership scenario, each patient pays $25 per month directly to the doctor on an annual membership contract. Then the patient pays $10 per doctor visit without any additional charges. These are the actual costs of an After Hours Medical membership.

When only seeing a doctor four times a year without any more visits to other health facilities, ERs, or hospitals, the following table summarizes what the 2,000 patients have to pay out of pocket in each of the two scenarios.

Here is a summary of the comparison of the two scenarios for visiting a doctor just four times a year:

Total Patients' Responsibilities	Health Insurance	Medical Membership
Monthly fee	Monthly Premium to Insurance	Monthly Fee to Doctor
For 2,000 patients	$1,200,000/month $14.4 million/year (2,000 x $600/mo x 12 mo)	$50,000/month $600,000/year (2,000 x $25/mo x 12 mo)
For each patient	$7,200/year ($600/mo x 12 mo)	$300/year ($25/mo x 12 mo)
Fee for 4 visits	Visit Fee ($500 Deductible)	Visit Fee ($10/visit)
For 2,000 patients	$960,000/year (2,000 x 4 x $120)	$80,000/year (2,000 x 4 x $10)
For each patient	$480/year (4 x $120)	$40 (4 x $10)

Table 2. Comparison of patient's responsibility in health insurance versus membership model.

In the health insurance scenario
- Each patient pays $7,200 annually for health insurance.
- This is a total of $14.4 million paid to the health insurance company by the 2,000 patients. It is put in reserve and not paid out to cover any of the four visits because none meet their $500 annual deductible.
- On top of the premium, each patient also has to pay an additional $480 to the doctor for the four visits, again, because the $500 deductible is not met.
- This $480 dollar annual payout by each patient is a savings of almost a million dollars ($960,000) for the insurance company thanks to the $500 deductible. That is, instead of insurance paying $960,000 to the doctor for the four visits, the patients have to pay this entire amount. *Imagine the savings for insurance plans with deductibles as high as $10,000!*

In the medical membership scenario
- Each patient pays only $300 a year, but directly to the doctor.
- This gives the doctor $600,000 per year, or $50,000 per month, to run his practice and to take care of 2,000 patients at four visits per patient per year.
- Each patient pays only $40 additionally for the four doctor visits.
- In this scenario, instead of collectively paying $14.4 million to the health insurance company for the four basic care visits it does not pay for anyway, the 2,000 patients only pay $600,000 to the doctor directly, saving $13.8 million for the patients for other necessities including, potentially, a major medical plan with a much lower premium that can be used in the event of a major medical crisis.

This comparison shows that it is possible to deliver four basic care visits to each of the 2,000 patients in a year with less than $1 million in cost, compared with the $14.4 million required by conventional insurance plans. One may argue that the way health insurance works is that the excess of the $14.4 million in this scenario, for example, is needed to help cover everyone's expense in case of unexpected loss (as well as covering those who are outside of this circle of 2,000 members.) However, I would argue that the premiums needed to cover these unexpected, major medical losses should be calculated based on major medical losses only, not to include basic medical care needs, which are taken care of by the membership program.

This comparison uses a hypothetically perfect medical practice. It compares one extreme scenario to another whereas reality can be anywhere in between, depending on various factors such as the health risk of patients in the practice—the less healthy will likely warrant more visits and higher chances for advanced care needs. Nevertheless, the point here is that we can help bring down healthcare costs and keep them low ourselves by working with our doctors directly and prepaying them using a capitation model.

The scenarios discussed here do not suggest that anyone should substitute a membership plan for their health insurance plan—doing so would not fulfill the requirements of Obamacare. It merely demonstrates how much money can be saved if the medical membership model is used to pay for basic medical care when compared to using a $2,000 to $10,000 high-deductible health plan for the same visits. Most importantly, it is crucial for the reader to know that this book suggests that the medical membership model be used *in conjunction with* health insurance plans to reduce medical care costs and insurance premiums while maintaining full health coverage. Under this proposal, insurance funds, which are increased by the Obamacare mandate, are not depleted and insurance premiums may not go up. This winning combination will happen only if we step up and build medical membership practices with our doctors nationwide. Lastly, imagine the growth of our membership model, and its cost savings, were Congress to incentivize nationwide implementation. What if this became part of the Affordable Healthcare Act?

Here is the solution: As shown in Figure 1, The solution to restore balanced healthcare dynamics, at the end of this chapter, imagine that just half of these savings are used to buy a health insurance (1) to cover major medical events only. Patients pocket the other half of the savings (2) while meeting their basic care needs with the medical membership program. (3) This combination would provide complete healthcare coverage for both basic care (4) and advanced care (5) at a much lower cost. Please refer to figure 1 at the end of this chapter.

Make Health Insurance "True Insurance"

The emerging availability of capitated medical practices that bypass insurance billing to take care of expected, basic medical care will make our current high-deductible health insurance plans obsolete. It will usher in more suitable health insurance plans like our car insurance—low premium plans designed to cover only major medical events that require expensive, specialized care. Just as car insurance does not pay for oil changes, health insurance should not pay for services that are equivalent to oil changes.

Medically speaking, routine services would include checkups, maintenance of chronic medical problems (such as heart disease and diabetes), and even minor illnesses and minor injuries that are a part of normal life, such as strep throat, simple broken bones, or the like. Once expected, routine healthcare services are widely provided under a capitation model by basic care doctors—providers who compete with one another by increasing quality and decreasing prices—then the costs of covering basic care needs will become even more affordable than they are now.

Basic care membership plans will leave health insurance funds to cover only catastrophic needs through major-medical-only health plans that comply with the requirements of Obamacare and work effectively in concert (and without legal hassles) with capitated medical membership programs. The beauty of these new major-medical-only insurance plans is that their premiums will be much lower and more affordable than the high-deductible health plans currently available on the market.

Supporters of our current health insurance plans may think that we are doing the right thing by increasingly purchasing high-deductible (and hence lower premium) health plans and using them in case of unexpected events or major medical catastrophe. Unhappily, these supporters do not see that high-deductible plans do not work in the long run. Time and again out-of-pocket expenses overtake a family's or individual's ability to pay. Again, look at the increasing medical bankruptcy in Massachusetts ever since the healthcare mandate took effect in 2006. After all, who can afford an unexpected payout of $2,500 to $10,000, potentially repeated across multiple years, in the event of an illness such as cancer?

When Americans are offered a product by their insurance companies that covers only advanced care and major medical needs that are above and beyond the scope of their capitated basic care provider, one that offers a significant saving, they will stand up and take note. As long as this product has a manageable premium, like that which they currently pay for their cars, then Americans will buy this product in droves and have their basic medical care needs met through cost-conscious capitated medical providers. Finally, both advanced care and basic care will be covered at prices families can more easily afford.

Let's do the math for another scenario in which an individual can experience significant savings by purchasing the combination of a medical membership plan and a major-medical-only insurance plan. Compare this scenario to paying for the typical $2,500 deductible plan that is popular at the writing of this book, as illustrated in Table 3 below.

	Scenario 1 Health insurance plan	Scenario 2 Major medical insurance plan with medical membership	
	$2,500 Deductible Health Plan	Major Medical only	After Hours Medical Medical Membership
Monthly Premium	$194*	$65**	$25
Per Visit Fee (est)	$120	none	$10
Annual Premium	$2,328	$720	$300
Fee for 4 Visits (est)	$480	none	$40
Total Annual Cost	$2,808	$1,060	
Annual Saving		$1,748 (62% saving)	

Table 3 shows the annual and monthly cost savings from using a medical membership plan for basic care, in conjunction with a major-medical-only insurance plan that does not cover basic care. *The $194 premium is from www.ehealthinsurance.com for a healthy 45-year-old male. **The $60 premium is an actual sample of what one of my editors paid in the late 1980's for a "managed major medical" health insurance plan available at that time.

This person can save $1,748 per year, or 62%, and is able to go to the doctor four times. Furthermore, the person will be able to put their premium savings into a tax-exempt Health Savings Account (HSA) that will serve them in the event they are forced to use their major-medical-only plan. If the person stays healthy and does not have any major medical events, they will see a similar saving accumulate every year and will eventually be able to have enough funds set aside to cover the costs that a major medical event could incur.

Furthermore, that person is covered in the event of medical catastrophe, or any medical event for which their capitated basic care provider would be unable to provide adequate care. There is no risk of financial insolvency and no temptation to avoid seeing a doctor for minor symptoms that could develop into a major illness if left untreated.

Restoring Competition, the Second Key

The act of combining a capitation plan for basic care with a health insurance plan that covers major medical events, in such a way that is compliant with Obamacare, could result in the disappearance of high-deductible health plans whose premiums are increasingly cost prohibitive and are driving Americans to bankruptcy. This will create a new area of competition among health insurance companies—the design, creation, and sale of major-medical-only health plans.

Competition is exactly what is missing among health insurance giants. This emerging, cutting-edge arena of competition offers a new point of entry that start-up health insurance companies can use to break into the health insurance market. This is the second key that Obamacare is missing in order to make healthcare reform successful—the restoration of free-market competition.

Creating an opportunity for start-up companies to enter the market will potentially bring down health insurance premiums. Imagine adding this to on top of the Obamacare limitation of 15% to 20% profit for insurance companies.

Nationwide there are dozens of new nonprofit health plans created under Obamacare's Consumer Operated and Oriented Plan Program (CO-OP). Much like credit unions, these health insurance co-ops are governed by the very members they insure and all profits are reinvested to improve care or lower premiums. Members will be able to elect the officers who run their co-op each year and in this way ensure that their co-ops continue to operate in their best interests—welcome, long-overdue, and revolutionary change.

My local co-op in Utah is Arches Health Plan, Inc. Some states have more than one, and some have none as this book goes to print. Hopefully start-up health insurance companies like Arches will seek competitive advantage by offering innovative new major-medical-only plans with low premiums suitable for my patients and all patients of capitated medical membership programs. If they do, they will accelerate the healthcare revolution.

However, as long as the The McCarran-Ferguson Act still shields giant insurance companies from federal antitrust laws, they will likely continue to behave in a monopolistic manner and attempt to squash competition and especially our new nonprofit co-ops. Unfortunately there are signs this has already begun in markets where co-ops have sprung up and giant health insurance companies have rolled out predatory pricing in the form of artificially low premiums for 2014. Low premiums are good news for consumers in the short term, but bad news in the long term if our nonprofit co-ops go out of business—if they do, the giants won't leave their rates low for long.

The emerging need for innovative, low-cost medical membership programs working in tandem with major-medical-only plans will encourage basic care providers and certain specialists to design and develop capitation plans of their own, thereby creating new competition among medical practices as discussed earlier. At least competition among providers will not be adversely affected by the The McCarran-Ferguson Act, which has enabled so many insurance companies to become monopolies in their given geographic markets.

When the competition for capitation plans for basic medical care increases in the market, what kind of savings could we have then? Who would be in control of the healthcare dollar at that point? That's right, you and me, consumers and medical providers, would finally be in control of the healthcare dollar. Some control is already in our hands because we eliminate the middleman and there's competition among capitation plans to help keep prices down.

Finally, the two key components missing in Obamacare have now been taken care of: 1) lack of control of medical care costs and 2) lack of competition among health insurance companies, as well as healthcare providers. We are now well on our way to working together to accept, create, and participate in capitation plans for basic medical care, and these programs now exist throughout our country. The healthcare revolution has begun.

Restoring the Past

Imagine your doctor getting paid ahead of time on a monthly basis. The doctor does not have to bill insurance, fight their denial, get paid several months later, or be told to bill you for the rest of the balance because you now have a deductible that you must meet.

Imagine you and other patients paying enough monthly to keep your doctor in business and cover the practice's overhead expenses. You will no longer see the practice billing you or your insurance for extra procedures.

Imagine that the much lower cost of prepaying your doctor, plus the much lower premium of a major-medical-only plan, can save you, your family, and your employer hundreds of dollars per month.

Imagine that you found your doctor and his capitated program because you have price-shopped and quality-shopped all of the capitated practices and chosen the membership program best for you. You can now call your doctor for a refill of your thyroid medication. If he has previously seen you on several occasions and knows your medical history, then will no longer have to insist that you must come in for a visit so he can run tests and bill your health insurance before refilling your prescription.

Imagine that because you and other patients have prepaid your doctor and kept him in business, you've freed him to follow the protocols of sound standard medical care and to control costs as doctors traditionally have in the United States. You've freed your doctor to simply do what's best for you, his patient.

As a member of his clinic, you can call him for questions and you will not hesitate to go in for regular checkups, regular maintenance of chronic conditions, and for minor problems to keep you healthy and out of hospitals. You also know that if you have to be in a hospital for a major health problem, you have the major-medical-only insurance to help cover that cost already.

Now you are no longer anxious as a consumer because you have a sense of control over your health, its related finance, and what to do in the event of a health catastrophe.

You may want to imagine even further a similar turn-around of hospitals, HMOs, and healthcare conglomerates. What if they change their fee-for-service model to more something more innovative and creative, perhaps even a capitation model that works for their systems by delivering advanced medical care under capitation and accepting the same capitation on their profits that Obamacare now places on insurance companies.

Finally, the True Purpose of Health Insurance

The original objective of buying health insurance coverage has been truly and soundly defeated by our present healthcare system. If you aren't already, you should be wondering why we have been coerced into paying so much for something that is supposed to provide care and financial security but that ends up costing us a fortune and landing so many of us in bankruptcy court.

Obamacare is a great start for a turnaround. It is paving the way but, on its own, will fail. Consumers and healthcare providers need to work together to provide the missing keys necessary to its health. The Obama Administration will have to tweak the Affordable Healthcare Act, but that's no problem because it's always expressed a willingness to do so.

Health insurance companies will have to create new and more affordable products to work with our own capitation plans.

We must all work to modify our healthcare system so that it promotes wellness and prevention as its main focus instead of excessive profit. Basic medical care should be provided at an affordable, capitated price by medical practices while keeping current private health insurers in the market, providing us with life-saving services through major medical plans that cover medical events not covered by basic medical membership plans.

In the end, individuals, families, employers, and employees will be able to regain control of their health and its related finances and prevent the demise of our healthcare system.

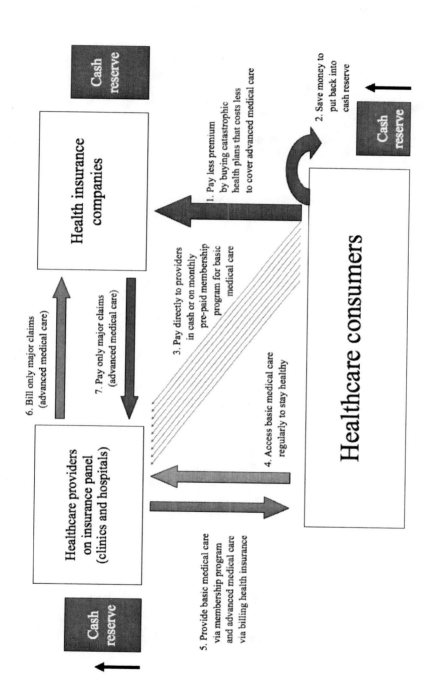

Figure 1. The solution to restore balanced healthcare dynamics.

Seven

Chapter 7
Medical Membership

So far I have examined the risks to our private healthcare system. In Chapter 5 I pointed out the root cause of dysfunction in our system, and in Chapter 6 I proposed a solution to keep our private healthcare system alive—capitation to control costs and foster competition that will help lower health insurance premiums.

This chapter talks specifically about one kind of capitation model, the medical membership program, and how practices nationwide can implement some version of it that suits their circumstances. The last chapter of this book will explain how such programs can complement Obamacare and help save our private healthcare system.

How It Originated in My Clinics

When the economy started to go downhill in 2008, my medical providers started to notice decreasing patient visits in the evenings. Upon interviewing our patients, we discovered that when they began to feel unwell they did not want to pay out of pocket for an after-work doctor visit, sometimes because they had lost their health insurance coverage. Instead many of them would stop by the pharmacy on their way home and pick up an over-the-counter medication and hope to sleep off their illnesses. When they did not get better the next morning, they would come into our clinics for medical care. Often by the time we saw them their illnesses had advanced to the point where they had to miss more work than they would have had they come in earlier. Likewise a few of them had to be referred to ERs, hospitals, or specialists for more costly medical care.

This observation prompted me to imagine a program that might allow my patients to come in for medical care at a lower rate that would help them recover more quickly and with fewer complications. I thought of a membership program similar to that of a gym membership where a monthly fee is enough to cover the cost of the gym and its profit, while allowing members to use it as frequently as they want to stay fit and healthy.

Initially I thought of avoiding a fee for each visit just like a gym but then quickly imagined the many potential pitfalls of a medical clinic without per-visit fees. Then I thought of Costco, where members can buy high-quality goods at discount prices (when compared to other typical retail stores), and considered charging for every medical procedure performed but at a discounted price. The tediousness of tracking and handling various prices, however, made me want to just keep things simple by going with one fee that represented a discount price for an entire visit, no matter how many procedures were performed. I finally decided to create a medical membership program that collects a monthly fee plus a modest fee for each visit, both fees being affordable enough for patients while still sufficient to cover our costs of operation with a reasonable profit.

I then encountered two challenges: legal requirements and determining the right prices.

First, I had heard that providing medical care for a monthly fee could be viewed as operating an insurance plan, and that a few years prior a doctor in New York "got in trouble with the law" for doing it. Luckily I found out that Utah laws regulating such programs were not prohibitive. The business model of offering discount medical services for a monthly fee falls under the laws governing medical discount programs in the state of Utah, not under health insurance regulation. Excited, I proceeded to build the program.

Second, I had to price my new membership product. In September 2009

I contacted a local actuarial firm that specializes in pricing plans for health insurance companies and learned of the enormous fees they would charge me for coming up with just two numbers: how much to charge per month and how much to charge per visit. Their hourly billing rate was $520 per hour with a $10,000 retainer. I decided to forgo the actuary and just go with my gut instinct to charge $49 per month per person and $5 per visit, and it worked.

After a couple of years in business and gathering data, I was able to lower the monthly fee to $25 per person per month and increase the per-visit fee from $5 to $10 just to cover operating costs and a reasonable profit. When people heard about my program they often thought it was too good to be true.

Curious, I researched our healthcare history and learned that my program was not anything new or innovative. In fact it was how our private health insurance industry started in 1929 when Dr. Michael Shadid created the first prepaid medical membership model in the United States.

After further research, interviews with patients and healthcare providers, and analysis of what I experienced firsthand as a doctor for 15 years, I was able to understand why the public thinks healthcare has to be expensive in order to be effective. Along the way I also discovered how we can work together to fix our broken healthcare system.

Capitation Is the Key

My capitated medical membership program is more effective from a cost and accessibility standpoint than our current health insurance for delivering basic medical care. Capitated models cover the expense of running a business, while offering a fair allowance for profit and preventing runaway costs and excessive profits. The capitation model should be applied to all businesses that provide services essential to life and health so that they remain accessible and affordable to everyone.

The capitation model is the opposite of what we have now—one with hidden costs and obscured prices that allows conglomerates and providers to gain unlimited profit from the business of keeping people alive and healthy.

A capitation model, medical membership being the most affordable, is what we can create and promote together in order to extend healthcare to more people and to reduce the use of unnecessary, expensive advanced resources. It is a way that medical providers and patients can work together directly to contain costs and bypass the middlemen. It is a sure way to provide basic medical care at a reasonable, transparent price. It is a sure way to reserve health insurance for major medical catastrophes just like car insurance is used only for unexpected losses. Finally, because of its upcoming popularity and its effectiveness in reducing costs, capitation is a sure way to establish a return to healthy market competition. In other words capitation is a good fit with the American free-enterprise system.

Why Does Medical Membership Work?

Medical membership can significantly reduce the costs of basic medical care when compared with health insurance plans. There's no need to involve a middleman in something that you and your basic care doctors can mutually agree to take care of together at a much lower cost. As previously shown in the hypothetical example comparing the health insurance model to the medical membership model, the membership model demonstrates that basic medical care is not expensive and can be taken care of at a much lower price than it is currently offered to most Americans. At the same time, medical membership covers the cost of running a medical practice.

Basic Healthcare Is Not Expensive

I am just amazed at all the comments I have received when people learned that membership in my clinic costs only $25 per month and $10 per visit. A quick survey of my medical membership program from a group of business owners yielded the following comments:

"You're crazy." – 3 people
"Too good to be true." – 3 people
"What's the catch?" – 21 people

These comments suggest that the general public believes healthcare is expensive and necessarily so. Without separating the prices for basic care (taking care of sore throat care, for example) from advanced care (taking out an appendix, for example), the way we separating the cost for an oil change from the cost for collision repair in the car insurance industry, it could very well be considered necessarily expensive.

Contrary to what most Americans believe, when basic care is separated from advanced care, healthcare in general is not expensive. As stated before, Wendall Potter talks about how he spent almost twenty years of his life as a public relations spokesperson leading insurance campaigns designed to make Americans believe that they could not live safely without health insurance coverage. These campaigns have instilled in the American mind that healthcare is an *expensive inevitability*. Health insurance representatives have championed the notion that the high costs of healthcare are justified, necessary, and even inevitable.

It is amazing how often people say "I can't see a doctor for my problem until I have health insurance." People automatically believe seeing a doctor is prohibitively expensive without insurance. Consequently many people in this country, including some doctors themselves, are surprised and skeptical when encountering clinics like mine. As long as we believe what large health insurance companies want us to believe, healthcare costs will remain high and become unaffordable for a growing number of Americans—with or without Obamacare.

As discussed at the beginning of Chapter 2, advanced medical care is much more expensive than basic medical care. This is because it involves use of specialized, expensive tools such as CT scans, MRI scans, operating room equipment and because it requires specialized facilities such as ERs, surgical centers, and hospitals.

Basic medical care, on the other hand, involves diagnosing and treating basic illnesses and injuries by using history and examination skills, as well as stethoscopes and prescription pads, blood tests, and a few other basic diagnostic tools.

Most medical conditions can be taken care of by basic care providers in their clinics and will never need to be referred to ERs, specialists, or to hospitals for further workup and treatment. Because of this, and because basic medical care is low cost, our overall healthcare costs should never be as high as they are today and can be contained by implementing capitation structures with   medical membership programs being the easiest, most effective, and quickest to set up.

Basic Care Medical Practices Have Fixed Costs

Because there are limited numbers of procedures that a basic care doctor can do in their clinic, and because most of the patients can be cared for without these procedures, a basic care doctor's office will usually have fixed costs with only small additional variable costs.

Dr. Brian R. Forrest in Apex, North Carolina, has one of the lowest-operating-cost cash clinics I have ever seen. He shared his annual operation costs openly on the internet. With his current patient base (probably close to two thousand patients), he claims that he sees about 16 patients a day, works 5 days a week, and that his costs are low.

Annual fixed costs

Medical Assistant salary (36 hours/week)	$31,500
Malpractice insurance	$10,500
Rent (he owns his own building)	monthly mortgage payment
Utilities	$5,250

Annual variable costs

Charges for tests by outside lab	$22,500
Medical supplies	$9,500
Miscellaneous (office supplies, internet, etc.)	$2,750

Total annual costs, fixed and variable	$82,000

Although total variable costs goes up if more patients come through the clinic's door, the average cost per patient will be a fixed, predictable amount for the most part, which can be seen as a fixed cost and usually covers the majority of expenses.

A typical basic care doctor works from 9 to 5, four to five days a week and can see up to 40 patients a day. No matter if the doctor has to see 10 patients or 30 patients a day, the cost is the same. The doctor has to pay the same rent and the same staff salary if they are working from open to close no matter how many patients are seen. These are his fixed costs.

Costs vary when the doctor perform procedures such as giving a shot or supplying breathing treatment for pneumonia, as opposed to just writing a prescription for an antibiotic to treat a sinus infection. The variable costs are for supplies—the shot and the breathing treatment, but these aren't so expensive so total remain relatively low, with little variation from month to month.

Membership programs work because, on average, the monthly fee covers all of the fixed costs and some of the variable costs, while the percentage of visits by a given patient population is manageable on the average and does not overwhelm the clinic. The doctors offering the membership programs will only have to charge enough monthly membership fees from everyone in that given population to produce a monthly income that is adequate to cover all the fixed costs and some of the variable costs of the operation and a moderate take-home wage for the doctor who is often the owner.

A typical family doctor usually is comfortable with seeing 15 to 20 patients a day. This rate is an ideal for family doctors because they can spend 20 to 30 minutes per patient visit, which is a lot better than modern doctors who bill health insurance and have to see about 30 to 40 patients a day to stay in business and be profitable. Doctors with their own membership programs can control and minimize the number of visits per day, so they can spend more time on each patient, optimize their medical care, and keep them healthy so they don't have to visit the clinic often. In this way a membership program has the potential for a family doctor to see fewer than 20 patients per day, spend more time with each, work 5 days a week, and still take home a reasonable salary. It all depends on how effectively the doctor and the membership program works. A great example is that of Dr. Forrest's practice. The fixed costs and variable costs for running his practice total $82,000 annually. With 2,000 patients to care for, he need see only an average of 16 patients per day. If one takes another step further and calculates the required monthly fee if his practice were to become a member clinic, he will only require less than $4 per month per member to cover the costs of running his practice!

$82,000 / 12 months / 2,000 patients

This example shows that a practice with operating costs and number of patients like that of Dr. Foster can clearly become a viable medical membership clinic.

Members Usage Is Manageable

In contemplating a new membership practice program, we typically fear that members might overuse their benefits, overwhelm the clinic, and increase its cost of operation. This scenario can be avoided by creating a reasonable agreement between members and providers. We'll discuss agreements in detail below. Fears aside, patient *usage*—the percentage of patient members who actually use the clinic in a given time period—will be relatively constant, at least in my experience.

Usage varies from one population to another and tends to increase during influenza season. For example, usage in a relatively healthy part of a large city will be less than that of another group in other parts of the same city. Each population and geographical area will have its own relatively steady usage rates depending on various characteristics of that population such as age, gender, medical risk factors, social risk factors—cigarette use, alcohol use, occupational exposure, etc. As each membership program is developed, monitoring usage and adjusting membership agreements and prices is the key to controlling practice costs and profit margins.

Variation within each patient population makes it important for a new membership program to set its membership fees and agreement with its members carefully and conservatively, that is, *higher at the beginning* in order to contain costs. Then as the membership program grows and matures, usage data can inform adjustment to fees and agreement terms to optimize profitability and patient affordability.

Membership Agreements

Just like any membership organization, mutual agreements need to be in place, understood, and accepted by all parties. Instead of one party claiming value over the other party, where one side wins while putting the other side at a disadvantage, a membership agreement needs to be "value creating." The agreement touches on areas of fees, benefits, and other *what-ifs*. Each membership agreement needs to create value for both parties, resulting in a fair exchange of medical benefits and payments. The best thing about creating a mutually beneficial agreement is that it is free of control from insurance, hospitals, and all other entities and thus puts control into the hands of practitioners and patients. The agreement just has to be in compliance with regulations for each state and should be prepared by legal counsel.

Here are some examples of areas of agreement that a membership program can draft to create value and protect the interests of both parties.

1. There should be a minimum membership commitment term of 6 to 12 months.

If the term were month to month, members could join the program during the months that they have medical need and drop out during the other months. Episodic use does not allow sufficient income generation from the months of no use to offset visit costs. So the idea of intermittent month-to-month payments cannot meet the two goals of keeping the business viable financially and keeping the costs down for all members. A minimum commitment of 6 to 12 months makes it attractive enough for patients to become members and also financially feasible for the doctor to take care of each member for $150 to $300. Each practice should adjust enrollment terms and rates to suit its circumstances. I caution that none of these changes should take place without dialogue with the members, and all changes should take into account competition from other capitation programs.

2. The membership program may create its own stipulations for accepting members or discharging members.

A practice that is new and wants to attract as many members as possible may elect not to have any screening requirement or any patient discharging rules. On the other hand, a practice that is full may put in place certain requirements for accepting new members. For example, a pain management clinic may have stricter requirements for patients to stay on the membership roster to help safeguard against the abuse of prescription drugs. The point here is that a practice can be as creative as it wants in order to make it work for both parties. But in general, a membership practice can make its own determination whether to accept new patients, and whom it will discharge just like any other non-membership or fee-for-service medical practice.

3. The doctors of the membership program reserve the right to refer any patients to other doctors, to other specialists, to emergency rooms, to hospitals, and to other facilities.

This allows the program to provide a reasonable standard of care and avoid any undue obligation to care for illnesses that go beyond their scope of training and experience, as any other non-membership or fee-for-service medical practices would. If a specialist offers a membership program, then the specialist will be able to do more for the patient in that specialized field than a family doctor can, therefore extending more benefit coverage in that field.

4. The program does not cover services rendered at other facilities outside of its practice.

Because it is not a health insurance plan, this requirement makes it clear that outside services are not the financial obligation of the program because the program simply cannot control the actions and the costs of outside entities. For example, if an MRI is indicated for back pain, then it needs to be performed at an outside MRI clinic that is probably not part of the program. The same goes for a member with a heart attack who needs to be sent to an ER for further evaluation. The cost of an ambulance ride to the ER and the ER care would not be covered by the program. (This is where a major medical insurance plan comes in.)

5. A cancellation fee must be assessed if the membership is cancelled prior to the end of the agreed term.

This helps discourage members from receiving services and then canceling, a financial burden upon the program and other members. Notwithstanding, some states require that members must be able to cancel within a certain days of joining a program.

6. Monthly membership fees must be made by automatic credit card charge or direct withdrawal from bank accounts.

Ongoing payment by members without invoicing may be necessary in order to avoid the cost burden of billing and following up on nonpayments. The only way this program can work is if the funds to sustain it come into the practice without interruption. Ideally some members may wish to pay a lump sum in advance.

These are examples of terms that should be agreed by the two parties in order for a membership program to work. Each membership program can be creative in deriving their standard agreement while meeting the program's ongoing objectives of financial viability and cost control. Each practice and each patient population will have different needs as membership programs are developed throughout the United States. These rules are necessary for the wellbeing and the profitability of the programs as well as the affordability and availability of medical care given to their members.

Medical Membership for Specialists

Conceptually and practically most specialist doctors are no different than family doctors. They both see their patients and perform procedures. A family doctor sees patients in their clinic and performs procedures such as strep test, immunization shots, x-rays, etc. A specialist also sees patients in their clinic and performs procedures such as burning warts for a dermatologist; trigger point injections for a pain specialist; taking out tonsils in an OR for an ENT specialist; or doing a heart bypass for a cardiothoracic surgeon. Medical memberships will work for some specialist, if not *most*, just as well as they do for family doctors.

Another area family doctors and many specialists have in common is that they both have fixed expenses for maintaining their private practices (except for hospital-based specialists who may not have offices of their own). Fixed expenses allow the calculation of a monthly membership fee to support the practice's operation. Many specialists, therefore, should be able to create medical membership programs of their own just like that of a family doctor. They can create their own program by basing their monthly membership fee on the monthly fixed costs of running their practice. They may charge higher rates than family doctors charge due to the complexity and the increased costs associated with their specialized procedures. The discounted price for each procedure may vary depending on the cost of its necessary supply, the length of time it takes, its level of difficulty, and the amount of training required in school to acquire the skill to perform the procedure.

As an example, a family doctor may charge $30 a month, $10 a visit, and $3 for a strep test (which is reimbursed at $12 by Medicare), whereas an endocrinologist (who mainly maintains diabetes and thyroid diseases, especially difficult cases) may charge the same $30 a month and $10 per visit fee, but $50 to perform a needle biopsy procedure of a thyroid (which is reimbursed at $146 by Medicare). Each doctor may have a 2,000–patient base so that the total monthly membership revenue will cover the monthly operating costs, while procedure fees cover the variable costs that come with supply usage and extra education for becoming an expert in doing a needle biopsy of the thyroid.

If an endocrinologist says that he only has 1,000 or 500 patients with advanced disease that are more difficult to take care of, and that the $30 monthly fee is not enough to cover his operating costs, then he has liberty to adjust his rate to cover his fixed costs simply because he is not being controlled by a third party. The specialist may argue that his monthly fee is higher than family doctors because specialist services cost more, longer training was needed to become a specialist, or that he is the only specialist in town to take care of more difficult patients with advanced diseases. My suggestion that specialists charge more than family doctors may sound exploitive, but this is in keeping with longstanding practice and the tenets of our free enterprise system in which prices are higher when the demand is high and the supply is low.

Other examples of specialists who can easily set up medical membership programs are pain management doctors, nephrologists, psychiatrists, dermatologists, or ophthalmologists, like Dr. David Masihdas, OD in Salt Lake City who has a membership program of his own.

As for specialists who perform procedures that are episodic and require operating rooms or hospitals, such as cardiologists (who use cardiac catheterization labs), general surgeons, and orthopedic surgeons, a medical membership program may not be feasible. These procedures should then be covered by a major-medical-only plan. However, if specialists with such expensive procedures want to also make capitation available in their private practices, it can be done. They can simply make their procedure prices transparent and affordable. Then financing services are available to pay the doctors and accept monthly payments from patients.

However attractive a concept a medical membership program may be, it is not ideal for all doctors. Some physicians who are strictly hospital based, for example, will have no ability to create a membership program for their patients, including anesthesiologists, internal medicine hospitalists, and intensive care doctors who work exclusively in hospitals.

Developing medical memberships for medical practices, whether for basic care or advanced care, opens up a whole new frontier of competitive medicine. It will allow all types of primary care and most types of specialist doctors to step up, be creative, and design programs with various features and fee structures of their own. Healthy competition and free enterprise should result in high-quality services, lower costs, and the ability of consumers to freely choose the care they want and from whom they want to receive it.

How to Get Started

When to Add Membership Program to Your Practice

The time to start membership programs is now. There is no reason to wait. If you are a patient looking for a medical membership program, bring a copy of this book to your doctor or a doctor whom you would like to start a membership program.

If you are a family doctor with your own practice and find yourself waiting for more patients, then you have room to add a membership program. This will not only help your patients who have no insurance, but will also help spark the healthcare revolution needed to solve our current crisis. It will also give you additional income at little additional cost provided that you set your membership fees correctly. The start-up costs may not be much and the process does not take long depending on the laws of your state. Once it is set up, the revenue from the program becomes additional income, helping to defray the costs of an existing practice.

Delay in starting membership programs simply means delay in regaining control of our healthcare and allowing the momentum of increasing medical care costs and insurance premiums. Every clinic and every doctor in the states that allow it should add membership programs to their practices as soon as possible. Membership programs should be created and accepted nationwide as soon as, and as much as, possible in order for consumers and doctors to mend our broken healthcare system. The creation of a nationwide network of medical membership programs depends on the willingness and the cooperation of patients and doctors to work together to make it happen.

In the near future, when medical membership and discount programs become widely popular and accepted nationwide, medical clinics can be created and started up too cater to members only. Unlike catering to patients with health insurance plans where billing is costly and payments are delayed, member-only clinics receive revenue directly from members up front, allowing the clinics to budget and operate more effectively and efficiently. Imagine finding an area in a city where thousands of people will instantly join a start-up clinic as members. If 2,000 people join at start up and pay $25 per month per person, the clinic will have $50,000 in revenue per month right away not only to operate the clinic but to turn a profit. When a member-only clinic can start up and financially sustain itself entirely with member support, we will know that our healthcare revolution has succeeded. In the meantime, clinics will have to start membership programs as add-ons to their fee-for-service operations until they have enough members to make their clinics member-only. Or if they so choose, they can remain both membership and fee-for-service based, just like my After Hours Medical clinics.

Legal Requirements

A medical membership program is simply a practice that receives a monthly fee from its members who then receive medical services at discounted prices.

The first priority in setting up a membership program is to find out the legal requirements in your state for rendering medical services for flat monthly fees. Some states have laws that regard this practice as discounted medical care and have certain requirements that the clinics must follow to set up the program, as does the State of Utah. Other states regard this practice as health insurance and require the clinics to follow the same regulations that health insurance plans have to follow. Insurance regulations can be strict and expensive, making it difficult and sometimes impossible to operate a medical membership program.

It is advisable to have an attorney to assist in setting up your membership program to avoid legal pitfalls. Each membership program must comply with state law. Below are some examples of requirements for the states of Texas and New York.

Texas Requirements

1. Complete the registration form with the Texas Department of Insurance and pay the $1,000 registration fee.
2. Provide biographies for each board member, executive officer, and program operator.
3. Provide a $50,000 Surety Bond.
4. Provide the Texas Department of Insurance with copies of all contracts used with subscribers/enrollees and agreements between the program and any healthcare provider.
5. Provide a list of all those who market the discount program. The list of marketers must be updated with the state on a quarterly basis. The update should be emailed to TDI-DiscountHealth@tdi.texas.gov
6. A Summary from TDI can be found here: http://www.tdi.texas.gov/licensing/agent/DisHealthCarePr.html

New York Requirements

1. As of May 2011, New York does not directly regulate Health Discount Programs. Nevertheless, the New York attorney general's office has fined Family Care and Medadvantage $10,000 and $15,000, respectively, for advertising tactics that the Attorney General's office determined to be unfair business practices, likely not staying within the following guidelines.

2. At present, New York has merely published some "guidelines" related to medical and prescription discount cards. On a high level these guidelines look a lot like what is required by the Utah statutes:

   a. The program must use plain language.

   b. The program must not use deceptive advertising.

   c. The program must not imply that it is health insurance and disclose in writing that it is not health insurance.

   d. The program must provide a toll-free number at which the discount program can be reached.

   e. If telemarketing is used, the program must comply with all telemarketing rules.

   f. If fax solicitations are used, they too must be done only in compliance with law.

   g. The program should provide 30 days' advance written notice before any material changes are made.

   h. The program should have a formal dispute resolution process.

   i. The program should allow a member to terminate within 30 days of enrollment if they never use the discount services.

Fee Determination

The next step in setting up a membership program is to determine what the monthly fees and the discounted fee for each service should be. In doing so, each medical practice needs to know the monthly cost of running its practice, which consists of fixed costs and estimated variable costs. The monthly cost of running a practice will differ from one practice to another but it is the basis for determining the fees of the membership program for each practice. Practices with lower operating costs will be able to provide lower membership fees when compared to practices with higher operating costs, which is the ultimate goal of a medical membership program.

There are three types of fees: the monthly fee (membership fee); the discounted fee for the visit; and the discounted fee for additional treatments and procedures. The monthly fee usually takes care of the monthly fixed costs of running the medical practice, whereas the per-visit fee takes care of the variable costs. The fees for additional procedures should be transparent, provided on a "menu" which details the costs of such procedures like rapid strep test, x-ray, splinting, etc.

Fixed Costs

Fixed costs are easier to calculate if the medical practice has definite hours of operation and definite staffing requirements. For example, a family practice clinic that opens from 9 a.m. to 9 p.m. seven days a week and staffed consistently will have operating costs that are more fixed and easier to calculate than practices that depend on one doctor whose operating hours vary according to the number of patients scheduled, procedures he has to perform, commitments elsewhere, and absences or time off. Naturally clinics that have fixed costs and fewer variable costs will have an easier time calculating the monthly membership fee and will trend toward lower fees.

Once the monthly fixed cost of running the practice is determined, the total number of members needed to completely cover the monthly fixed cost can be determined by dividing the monthly cost by the monthly fee the clinic chooses to charge each member. Another important number is the monthly usage by members. Usage can be drawn from data in an established practice or estimated for a start-up. This number will come into focus as the program matures and fees may be adjusted accordingly. Based on my experience in my clinics, usage ranges from 20% to 40%, depending on the season.

Let's suppose that it costs $40,000 per month to run a medical clinic serving 1,000 members. That clinic will have to charge *at least* $40 per member per month (PMPM) to break even. If the practice wants to make $10,000 a month in profit, it will have to charge $50 PMPM...or enroll additional members. At 20% usage the clinic will have 200 visits per month or 50 visits per week. This is 10 patient visits per day if the clinic opens 5 days a week, or 7 visits per day if the clinic opens 7 days a week. If 20% happens to be the actual usage, then it is clear that the clinic can easily make its $50,000 per month income target with only 10 patient visits per day, opening only 5 days a week. The clinic can obviously handle more members or even lower its fees to make the program more affordable.

If we give it a worst-case scenario and increase usage from 20% to 40%, then the clinic can still easily take care of 20 visits per day for its 1,000 members and still open only 5 days a week while making $50,000 per month from monthly membership fees alone.

Variable Costs

Once members pay their monthly membership fees, they are entitled to receive medical services at discounted prices. This is similar to a health insurance plan agreeing to pay for these medical services, each with its own procedure code, at different fees. These fees vary from one health insurance plan to another. The main difference is that health insurance carriers are often third-parties who pay claims for their members to receive medical care from doctors and then take a cut for themselves via the premiums. In contrast, membership programs are created by doctors themselves to receive direct payment from patients for each procedure code (i.e., each service) at a discounted, transparent price without third-party overhead or profits.

Membership programs may elect to set their own discounted price for each procedure performed or simply roll common procedures into the office visit fee without extra charge. For example, an office visit level-III for a new patient, which can be billed to health plans at $100 and reimbursed at Medicare's rate of $70 (in Utah), may be given to members at a discounted price of $20. A strep test, which is reimbursed by health insurance plans at an average of $12 per test, may be given to members at a discounted price of $5 as these are reimbursed far more than warranted by Medicare, in addition to the $20 office visit fee. Alternately the practice can elect to set the office visit fee at $25 to $30 and include the rapid strep test, or any other procedures for that matter, without additional charge.

In addition to the charge for each office visit, charging additional discounted prices for various tests, treatments, and procedures is highly recommended and may be suitable for specialists whose procedures are more costly and whose operational costs are more variable. As an example, an ophthalmologist may elect to charge the same $20 to $30 PMPM as a family doctor, but then charge half of what Medicare would pay for a cataract surgery and other specialized procedure. If a new patient wants a cataract surgery at the discount price, they could become a member for $25 to $30 per month and commit to an annual contract. This may turn out to be the best deal for a patient needing cataract surgery in term of actual dollars spent, plus it enables them to have extensive follow-up at a reasonable cost. The main objective is the reduction and capitation of the cost for cataract surgery, although providing good care at a great price can be its own best advertising—patients are sure to spread the word.

Software Needed

Another start-up requirement is a software program that can host membership accounts, charge members' credit cards or bank accounts monthly, and determine if members are current with their monthly payments (or not) before being seen and receiving medical services. This can be done manually albeit laboriously. A practice can also use a CRM (customer relationship management) program to help track members and use Intuit QuickBooks®, or similar software, to generate monthly bills. Outside service companies that help manage memberships for health clubs or gyms can also be used for this purpose.

What about members whose accounts are not current? The answer is that the clinic can elect to handle such members however the clinic wants. Just like other clinics, large practices, and hospitals in traditional fee-of-service settings, what the clinic with membership chooses to do may vary from refusing care for outstanding balances to taking care of the patients first and then following up on the outstanding balances later. Such collection process may be part of the software or companies that health clubs and gyms use to maintain their membership and check their customers in at the time of service.

Ready... Launch!

Once the fees are set, the software is ready, and a license is in place, the clinic can start signing up members and taking care of them with the current staff, without having to increase staffing or change existing operational procedures—unless the number of members and their visits significantly increase down the road. At that time, the clinic should have enough revenue from membership fees to make appropriate changes to accommodate more members.

Once up and running, the clinic can either see their patients on a walk-in basis or on an appointment basis. Clinics that have finite operational hours may see their members needing medical services on a walk-in basis while clinics that have variable operational hours may elect to see their members by appointment only. Making appointments helps to control the cost of the clinic better and may be more suitable for family doctors.

Once membership programs are established and running extensively throughout the United States, one can imagine how readily consumers will access basic medical care to become healthier, reduce the need for costly advanced care, and help reduce their health insurance premiums. For graduates coming out of medical schools there will be less hesitation to become family doctors because the career and its prepaid income have now become financially viable only three years away from medical school graduation when compared to five years for specialists—an incentive that may help increase the number of primary care doctors, who can promote affordable healthcare for more Americans. It may also help decrease the number of graduates entering specialty fields and permit existing specialists to concentrate on patient care rather than trying to figure out how to survive, compete, and run profitable practices.

Eight

Chapter 8
Capitation Brings Revolution

By this time I hope I have adequately demonstrated that our private healthcare system is in crisis having allowed the cost of healthcare and health insurance to escalate, without cap in a profit-driven spiral between medical providers and insurance carriers.

I have also attempted to demonstrate that the key to controlling healthcare costs is to provide basic medical care under a capitated medical membership model that can keep everyone healthier for less money and will also keep medical practices prepaid and viable. This will, in turn, reduce the chances of depleting the health insurance funds now mandated by Obamacare, preserving those funds for major medical coverage. Along with capitation for basic care, the restoration of competition among insurance companies and the creation of competition among healthcare providers can further reduce health insurance premiums and deductibles, as well as reducing overall cost of medical care. I believe the best capitation method is the medical membership model that needs to be accepted by consumers and providers equally and incorporated into medical practices nationwide as soon as possible. This is something we can work together to accomplish.

This final chapter discusses how capitation, the key to preventing the demise of our private healthcare system, complements Obamacare and helps make the law work successfully in repairing our healthcare crisis.

Working with Obamacare

President Obama may not enjoy overwhelming support for his healthcare reform law, but he really should be applauded for at least two accomplishments that help pave the way for us to step in and improve US healthcare. First, the mandate requiring individuals to purchase, and requiring employers to provide, health insurance might be hard to swallow for many people. Nonetheless, it will certainly cause more funds to become available in the collective insurance pool to theoretically, and hopefully, cover medical care costs for everyone. Secondly, the cap on profits health insurance companies can take will help protect insurance reserves. Obamacare paves the way for successful healthcare reform.

Without our help Obamacare will not fix the American healthcare system. Increased insurance funds will be at risk of depletion by various means including "using it to cover everything," which will snowball into higher premiums and invite other negative outcomes discussed in this book.

Therefore, it is crucial that someone come up with a plan that complements Obamacare for real reform to take root. This someone may as well be you and me because no one else has our best interests at heart. This joint plan must protect insurance reserves from unnecessary and expensive procedures ordered and paid for beyond reasonable standards of medical care—and too often only for profit.

Our capitated solution could benefit from government incentives and thoughtful support by policymakers, but thankfully it does not require governmental intervention or billions of dollars or jumping through regulatory hoops, or even lobbying Congress. Our plan only requires us to step up to the plate and make it work. Our payoff is greater control of the US private healthcare system, our own health, and our finances. All it takes is for our doctors and medical practices to take advantage of the laws regulating discounted medical care in their states and add medical membership programs, then for us, average Americans, to embrace old-fashioned doctor-patient relationship building and join these programs.

When my medical membership program rolled out in September 2009, I thought everyone would jump on board immediately and take advantage of such affordable care. It made *so much sense* that people would want to save money. It didn't happen. The public was too set in their belief that health insurance is an essential part of life and a necessary evil—why else would people pay higher insurance premiums with higher out-of-pocket expenses for less care every year? This mindset has clouded their thinking for so long that better alternatives have been completely ignored.

Now it is getting to the point where enough of the public can see that they are being exploited by the healthcare system. They are ready for an alternatives and ready to take matters into their own hands.

Proper Use of Health Insurance: Major Medical Only

Individuals, families, small businesses, and large businesses need to shy away from purchasing costly high-deductible health plans when capitation plans for basic care become available. The graph below shows how obsolete a high-deductible plan looks beside a medical membership plan. Once the alternative of membership plans with their many advantages are widely understood, market forces will push health insurers to abandon high-deductible plans and offer major-medical-only plans with low deductibles. Since premiums for each plan are calculated based on coverage, a major-medical-only plan with limited coverage ought to have a lower premium than that of a high-deductible health plan that covers everything.

The diagram on the following page compares how much a patient would pay for medical care in two different scenarios. In the first scenario, using only a high-deductible health plan, the premium is much higher. It is calculated based on the entire spectrum of coverage, even for the portion that the member will have to pay on their own due to the deducible. Then when the member visits a doctor, they have no idea how much the visit will cost. In the second scenario, the premium is lower because it is calculated based only on coverage for major medical needs, and does not include basic medical care. Basic medical care is then managed by a medical membership program used in conjunction with a major-medical-only plan. The member

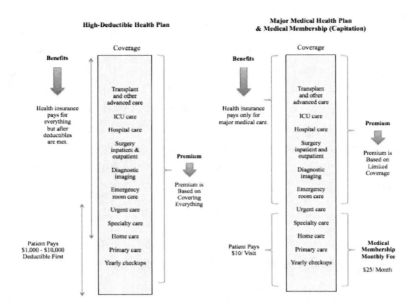

knows exactly how much each of the basic care visits will cost and knows that it will always be relatively affordable. In the meantime, the member has peace of mind knowing that any potential major medical problems will be taken care of by the health insurance plan that has been set aside for that purpose at a much more affordable premium.

Consumers will be searching for health plans that have major-medical-only coverage very soon, if they aren't already—rendering high deductible insurance plans obsolete. Such major-medical-only plans will cover procedures and treatments that are expensive but often needed unexpectedly, such as CT scans, MRI scans, major surgeries, hospitalizations, cancer treatments, organ transplants, etc. This is what I call the proper use of health insurance. These plans will become increasingly popular and in high demand starting in 2014 and 2015 when the Obamacare mandate takes full effect. Unfortunately, such major-medical-only plans will not meet the mandate requirement because they do not fulfill the "minimal essential coverage" required by the law. This is an area where our lawmakers can step up— such major-medical-only plans should be accepted by the mandate as long as they are coupled with medical membership plans to cover basic medical care needs.

An example of major-medical-only health plans is a group of "managed major medical" plans that were available in the 1980s but that have since disappeared. Such plans did not cover any regular doctor visits or any basic medical care. They would cover only major medical events and costly medical care. One of my editors, Susan, had such a plan when she was growing up in the 1980s. She paid $65 per month for a major medical plan that only covered medical emergencies and hospitalizations.

Table 1 below helps illustrate the savings in premiums and out-of-pocket costs between a traditional high-deductible plan and a major-medical-only plan coupled with a medical membership program:

	Scenario 1 Health insurance plan	Scenario 2 Major medical insurance plan with medical membership	
	$2,500 Deductible Health Plan	Major Medical only	After Hours Medical Medical Membership
Monthly Premium	$194*	$65**	$25
Per Visit Fee (est)	$120	none	$10
Annual Premium	$2,328	$720	$300
Fee for 4 Visits (est)	$480	none	$40
Total Annual Cost	$2,808	$1,060	
Annual Saving		$1,748 (62% saving)	

Table 1. This table compares the financial outcome of a scenario where a traditional high-deductible health plan is used alone to a scenario in which a combination of a major-medical-only health plan is used in conjunction with a medical membership program.

Suppose that Susan now pays $194 per month for a $2,500 deductible health plan with Blue Cross (an actual quote from www.ehealthinsurance. com for a single 45-year-old person). But she wants to go back to the 1980s and pay $65 per month for a "managed major medical" plan and use the medical membership program at After Hours Medical for $25 per month and $10 per visit. If she goes to the doctor 4 times a year, with an average reimbursement per visit of $120, Susan will save $1,748 or 62% in the first year while developing a valuable provider-relationship and enjoying peace of mind that comprehensive health care is both readily available and affordable.

Perfect for Family Doctors

As supported by my calculations in Chapter 7, it would be better for a family doctor to accept a dollar a day from all of his 2,000 patients each month basis than to use his own capital to operate his clinic and then wait for delayed payments from insurance carriers and patients—and hope to stay in business. There is little doubt that if a few doctors in every city were to develop and integrate medical membership into their practices, word will spread and more practices will follow.

Finally, member patients will readily go in for visits and checkups, resulting in better health and happier primary care doctors who are free to deliver medical care however they believe in order to produce the best outcome for both themselves and their patients. This may actually increase the number of primary care doctors over the years and solve the problem of our national shortage of primary care physicians.

What if our government were to offer incentives for doctors to create and maintain medical membership programs? Imagine an even more positive outcome with lower medical care costs and healthier Americans across the nation.

To help make this utopia of family medicine work for us all, consumers should contact their doctors and urge them to make medical membership programs available and then promote them by joining the programs. Doctors and medical practices should recognize and accept this new trend, as well as research the financial advantages over fee-for-service models wherein remittances are slow, cumbersome, and costly.

Medical membership in a family doctor's office is definitely a new but cost effective way of delivering medicine that can be set up quickly with little cost, while showing quicker results in both the doctors' business outcomes as well as their patients' health outcomes.

Healthcare Conglomerates

Many private medical practices now struggle to keep their businesses afloat. They have nowhere else to go, except to file bankruptcy, leave the country, retire, or join hospitals or healthcare conglomerates whose current goals are to maximize the fee-for-service method for profit generation.

Now that family doctors and specialty doctors have a better alternative to help sustain their practices, one that can be created quickly and without much capital investment, they do not have to surrender themselves to employment by corporations that will make them work even harder than they do now. Their freedom and the independence of their practices can continue.

In the process, hospitals and healthcare conglomerates will remain available for necessary major medical needs. Their expensive, high-tech resources will be reserved for referral of cases that truly need these resources just like back in the good old days when independent doctors used them infrequently and only when necessary. The practice of convenient referrals for costly medical procedures, and sometimes for unnecessary or unethical reasons, will greatly decrease. Family doctors and specialty doctors across the nation will remain independent, using whatever capitation model they choose and will not be under any employment pressure to increase usage of costly medical procedures.

Instead of pressuring medical providers for referrals, hospitals and healthcare conglomerates will have to work with—even court—capitated medical practices in their communities to earn their referral business. In doing so, they will demonstrate the respect that these medical professionals deserve and treat medicine as a way to provide life-enhancing care to consumers as opposed to using medicine to exploit them for excessive profit.

In Conclusion

In order to find the right answer to our current healthcare crisis, we need to ask the most fundamental question: What is the purpose of health insurance?

To consumers who buy health insurance, the purpose is to have payment coverage when seeking medical care to stay healthy (and to avoid the complications of serious untreated injury and illness, and even death) without significant financial strain.

To some of the other players in our private healthcare system who sell and receive payment from health insurance and who provide health insurance themselves, motives vary, but not generally in the interest of the consumers—leading to the root of the problem, the exploitive dynamic between providers and insurers.

At the end of the day, it all comes down to justice and fair play—receiving enough benefits from the product we spend so much on, especially when we are forced to buy it or else face legal consequences.

Joel Dickson posted the following comment as recently as July 12, 2013 in the Ogden, Utah *Standard-Examiner*:

I am an individual purchaser with a family health insurance plan that is a high-deductible plan with lower premiums and a $7,000 per year family deductible. On Aug. 1, 2011 the plan cost me $499 per month. On Aug. 1, 2012 the cost of the plan rose to $588 per month. On Aug. 1, 2013 the cost of the plan will rise to $726 per month. That is an increase of more than $2,700, or 22.5 percent per year………At current rates I have to pay $8,712 in premiums and $7,000 in deductibles, or nearly $16,000 annually before my insurance company pays for any of my family health care expenses. That is simply unaffordable and **represents 29 percent of Utah's average household income**, *which is approximately $55,000.*

Compare this to the situation in 1940s when an American family's average annual median income was $2,378, of which $148 was paid for medical expenses—only 6% of their income.

Clearly justice is not served to consumers in our day when they already pay so much in premiums and out-of-pocket fees. The goal is to have this 29% potential family health expenditure reduced to 6% as it was in the past.

There's no single problem in our dysfunctional healthcare system that we should pick out of a lineup; to do so would create new or worse problems. Instead it's the interplay among entities in our current healthcare system that has caused the healthcare mess we have now. Because the interplay involves everyone— consumers, providers, health insurers, and the government—no one entity can be expected to fix our healthcare problems and be successful. This is why Obamacare alone, representing the government in this dynamic, will not succeed at repairing our broken private healthcare system.

The solution requires all of us to step up to the plate and do whatever is necessary to repair the system as laid out in detail in Table 2 at the end of this chapter. In demanding affordable health insurance options and seeing to our basic health care in more effective ways, we will automatically enable our doctors to prosper in their fields of medicine without uncontrollable strain on their businesses. We will also allow insurance funds generated by government mandate to remain healthy and available to cover the legitimate, advanced healthcare costs for everyone.

Our government can go further in its effort to create effective healthcare reform. First, our government needs to redefine the "minimal essential benefits" in its reform law with more detail, as well as pass additional legislation to allow health insurance companies to design plans that cover only major medical issues so that health insurance premiums become, and stay, affordable. Of course this presumes that individuals holding such policies will have capitated basic care plans in place.

Second, our government needs to pass laws supporting the creation of medical membership programs nationwide. This will help resolve the issue of primary care doctor shortages, one of the reasons US medical care is become the most costly in the world without superior outcomes.

I hope that you and your family can now see the light at the end of the tunnel where a clear plan of action is awaiting all of us so we can bring the 29% household expenditure on healthcare down much closer to the 6% where it should really be. With this goal in sight, we will prevent the *demise of our healthcare*.

Important Attributes	Healthcare Providers	Consumers	Health Insurance Companies	Our Government
Medical membership: an innovative solution	Provide capitated medical membership programs for consumers.	Buy into medical membership programs.	Provide major-medical-only insurance products with low premiums and low deductibles.	Allow creation of major-medical-only insurance plans to be an acceptable part of the Obamacare mandate.
Medical membership, used in conjunction with health insurance plan: a cost-reduction strategy	For patients who have both insurance plans and medical membership programs, bill the insurance for major medical procedures and use medical membership programs for basic care—not using both plans for the same procedure.	Encourage your workplace to offer and subsidize a medical membership program in conjunction with major-medical-only insurance plan. Use medical membership for basic care to stay healthy in order to minimize the use of insurance.	Provide a variety of coverages for major-medical-only insurance plans for consumers who choose to buy into medical membership programs.	Allow the combination of major-medical-only insurance plans and medical membership programs to be an acceptable option under the Obamacare mandate.
Medical membership for prevention, health insurance for major medical catastrophe; a health-promoting strategy	Steer medical membership programs toward wellness and preventative medicine. Enhance doctor-patient relationship to reduce chances for major medical catastrophe.	Adhere to your doctor's wellness and preventative program. Accept that a reasonable standard of care might not include as many procedures, especially advanced procedures, as you have come to believe.	Provide wellness discounts for consumers who get regular checkups and are willing to use medical membership programs for basic medical needs instead of going to emergency rooms or hospitals first.	Educate the public about what reasonable standard of care looks like for common illnesses, so they do not seek out unnecessary procedures.
Standardization and accountability regarding basic care by medical membership programs	Membership providers should provide health data and various metrics to health insurance and the state government to ensure quality and effectiveness of their wellness and preventative programs.	Comply with wellness and preventative program by your membership doctor. Stop suing practices that provide a reasonable standard of care.	Recognize and reward practices with effective medical membership programs that prevent the insured from incurring expensive care at emergency rooms and hospitals.	Allow each state to create a governing body to monitor the profit margins of medical membership practitioners, their standards, and their quality as they do with insurance companies.
Standardization and accountability regarding advanced care by health insurance plans	Be willing to justify the use of extensive workup and advanced medical procedures within a reasonable standard of care for individuals whose symptoms warrant such.	Educate yourself and temper your expectations. Accept that a reasonable standard of care might not include as many advanced procedures as you have come to believe.	Monitor the use of advanced medical procedures and extreme price deviations. Report procedures that are out of the standard of care to the appropriate state or federal governing agencies.	Standardize the use of advanced major medical procedures. Outlaw the use of procedures for the purposes of revenue generation and increasing profit margins by medical practices, ERs, and hospitals.

Table 2. This table summarizes actionable items that all of us, insurance companies, and our government can step up and take ownership of in order to make healthcare available and affordable for everyone.

Bibliography

Bibliography

Accenture. (2012). Clinical transformation: New business models for a new era in healthcare. Retrieved August 25, 2013, from http://www.accenture. com/SiteCollectionDocuments/PDF/Accenture-Clinical-Transformation-New-Business-Models-for-a-New-Era-in-Healthcare.pdf#zoom=50

Alexander, A. & Neff, J. (2013, February 8). Lawsuit: Blue cross stifles competition. Charlotte Observer. Retrieved August 25, 2013, from http://charlotteobserve.com/2013/02/08/3842399/lawsuit-blue-cross-stifles-competition.html#.UilaYpWtg0x

American Medical Association. (2010, February 23). AMA study shows competition disappearing in the health insurance industry. Press Release. Retrieved September 5, 2013, from http://www.ama-assn.org/ama/pub/news/health-insurance-competiton.page

American Public Healthcare. (2012, August). Affordable care act overview. Retrieved September 5, 2013, from http://www.apha.org/advocacy/Health+Reform/ACAbasics/

Berry, E. (2011, August 15). Health plan profits coming before growth membership. Amednews.com. Retrieved September 5, 2013, from http://www.amednews.com/article/20110815/business/308159964/4/

Berry, E. (2008, May 19). Health plans say they'll risk losing members to protect profit margins. Amednews.com. Retrieved September 5, 2013, from http://www.amednews.com/article/20080519/business/305199998/1/

Bureau of Transportation Statistics (n.d.) Table 1-11: Number of U.S. aircraft, vehicles, vessels, and other conveyances. Department of Transportation. Retrieved August 25, 2013, from http://www.rita.dot.gov/bts/sites/rita.dot.gov.bts/files/publications/national_transporation_statistics/html/table_01_11.html

Care Cooperative Inc.. (2013). Appendectomy. Healthcare Blue Book. com. Retrieved September 5, 2013, from http://www.healthcarebluebook.com/page_Results.aspx?id=43&dataset=hosp&g=Apendectomy

Catlin, A., Cowan, C., Hartman, M. & Heffler, S. (2008, January). National health spending in 2006: A year of change for prescription drugs. HealthAffairs.org. Retrieved September 5, 2013, from http://content.healthaffairs.org/content/27/1/14.long

CBS News. (2009, February 11). COD = cash-only doctors. Associated Press. Retrieved August 25, 2013 from www.cbsnews.com/2100-204_162-610269.html

Cecere, D. (2009, September 17). New study finds 45,000 deaths annually linked to lack of health coverage: Uninsured, working-age Americans have 40 percent higher death risk than privately insured counterparts. In Harvard Gazette. Retrieved August 25, 2013, from http://news.harvard.edu/gazette/story/2009/09/new-study-finds-45000-deaths-annually-linked-to-lack-of-health-coverage/

Centers for Medicare and Medicaid. (2011). NHE fact sheet. Retrieved September 5, 2013, from http://www.cms.gov/Research-Data-and-Systems/Statistics-Trends-and-Reports/NationalHealthExpenddata/NHE-Fact-Sheet.html

Collins, S., Robertson, R., Garber, T. & Doty, M.M. (2013, April). Insuring the future: Current trends in health coverage and the effects of implementing the affordable care act: findings from the commonwealth fund biennial health insurance survey, 2012. Commonwealth Fund.org., Retrieved September 5, 2013, from http://www.commonwealthfund.org/~/media/Files/Publications/

Fund%20Report/2013/Apr/1681_Collins_insuring_future_biennial_
survey_2012_FINAL.pdf

Collins, S., Robertson, R., Garber, T. & Doty, M.M. (2012). Insuring the
future: Current trends in health coverage and the effects of implementing
the affordable care act. Commonwealth Fund.org., retrieved August 25, 2013
from http://www.commonwealthfund.org/Publications/Fund-Reports/2013/
Apr/Insuring-the-Future.aspx

Devereaux, P.J., Choi, P.T., Lacchetti, C., Weaver, B., Schunermann, H.J.,
Haines, T., et al. (2002, May 28). A systematic review and meta-analysis
of studies comparing mortality rates of private for-profit and private not-
for-profit hospitals. Canadian Medical Association Journal 166(11): 1396-
406. Retrieved on August 25, 2013, from http://www.ncbi.nlm.nih.gov/
pubmed/12054406

Doyle, D. (2013, February 2). Where your clients might be losing money in
their practices. Healthcare Billing and Management Association. Retrieved
September 5, 2013, from http://www.hbma.org/news/public-news/n_where-
your-clients-might-be-losing-money-in-their-practices

Elliot, V.S. (2012, August 14). Increase in physician practice mergers and
acquisitions expected to continue. Amednews.com. Retrieved August 25, 2013
from http://www.amednews.com/article/20120814/business/308149997/8/
Elliot, V.S. (2011, October 24). Residents' desire for hospital employment
poses recruiting challenge for practices. Amednews.com. Retrieved
August 25, 2013 from http://www.amednews.com/article/20111024/
business/310249968/1/

Fuhrmans, V. (2008, September 22). Consumers cut health spending, as
economic downturn takes toll. Wall Street Journal. Retrieved September 5,
2013, from http://online.wsj.com/article/SB122204987056661845.html

Furnas, B. & Buckwalter-Poza, R. (2009, June). Health care competition:
Insurance market domination leads to fewer choices. Center for American

Progress. Retrieved August 25, 2013, from http://www.americanprogress. org/issues/2009/06/pdf/health_competitiveness.pdf

Grande, D., Barg, F.K., Johnson, S. & Cannuscio, C.C. (2013 January/ Fedbruary). Life disruptions for midlife and older adults with high out-of-pocket health expenditures. Annals of Family Medicine 11(1) 37-42. Retrieved August 25, 2013 from http://annfammed.org/content/11/1/37.full
Health Cost Institute. (2013, May 15). New study tracks impact of aging on health costs. HCCI. Press Release. Retrieved September 5, 2013, from http://www.healthcostinstitute.org/2010report

Health Care for America Now. (2010, February). Health insurers break profit records as 2.7 million Americans lose coverage. Retrieved September 5, 2013, from http://hcfan.3cdn.net/a9ce29d3038ef8alel_dhm6b9q01.pdf

Health Grades Inc. (2013, May 7). Prevalence and incidence of acute appendicitis. rightdiagnosis.com. Retrieved September 9, 2013, from http:// www.rightdiagnosis.com/a/acute_appendicitis/prevalence.htm

Helfand, D. (2010, February 4). Anthem blue cross dramatically raising rates for Californians with individual health policies. Los Angeles Times. Retrieved September 5, 2013, from http://articles.latimes.com/2010/fen/04/ business/la-fi-insure-anthem5-2010feb5

Henry J. Kaiser Foundation (2011). Hospital emergency room visits per 1,000 population. Retrieved on August 25, 2013, from http://kff.org/other/ state-indicator/emergency-room-visits/#

Himmelstein, D., Woodhandler, S. & Almberg, M. (2011, March 8). Massachusetts reform hasn't stopped medical bankruptcies: Skimpy health insurance policies are likely culprit in continuing problem; findings indicate national reform law won't stop bankruptcies. Physicians for a National Health Program. Retrieved September 5, 2013, from http://www. pnhp.org/news/2011/march/massachusetts-reform-hasnt-stopped-medical-bankruptcies-harvard-study

How can hospitals afford to own physician practices. (2012, November 13). Trustee.knowledgebase.co. Retrieved August 25, 2013, from http://trustee.knowledgebase.co/article/white-paper--how-can-hospitals-afford-to-own-physician-practices-20.html

Horn, A., (2010). National shortage of primary care physicians felt locally. Spotlight on Health Summer 2010. CentraCare Health.com. Retrieved August 25, 2013, from http://www.centracare.com/community/spotlight/physician_shortage.html/

Kavilanz, P. (2013, April 26). Doctor. 'I gave up on health care in America'. CNN Money.com. Retrieved September 5, 2013, from http://money.cnn.com/2013/04/26/smallbusiness/doctor-quit-healthcare/index.html

Kavilanz, P. (2013, April 8). Doctors driven to bankruptcy. CNN Money.com. Retrieved September 5, 2013, from http://money.cnn.com/2013/04/08/smallbusiness/doctors-bankruptcy/index.html

Keehan, S., Sisko, A., Truffer, C., Smith, S., Cowan, C., Poisal, J., et al. (2008, February). Health spending projections through 2017: The baby-boom generation is coming to Medicare. HealthAffairs.org. Retrieved September 5, 2013, from http://content.healthaffairs.org/context/27/2/w145.abstract

Manoj, J. (2012, March 12). Doctors in private practices are now joining hospital staffs. Washington Post. Retrieved August 25, 2013 from http://articles.washingtonpost.com/2012-03-12/national/35448596_1_medicare-cuts-physician-practices-doctors

Marks, J.W. (2004). Prompt pay statutes for physicians' billing claims: An imperfect remedy for a systemic problem. Journal of Medical Practice Management. Retrieved September 5, 2013, from http://www.bmm-law.com/Images/Prompt_Pay_Statutes.pdf

Medical Group Management Association. (2012). Physician compensation and production survey 2012 report. www.mgma.com. Retrieved August 25, 2013, from http://www.mgma.com/store/Surveys-and-Benchmarking/Physician-Compensation-and-Production-Survey-2012-Report-Based-on-2011-Data-Print-Edition/

Merrit Hawkins. (2011). 2011 review of physician recruiting incentives: An overview of the salaries, bonuses, and other incentives customarily used to recruit physicians. MerritHawkins.com. Retrieved August 25, 2013, from http://www.merrithawkins.com/pdf/mha2011incentivesurvPDF.pdf

National Association of Community Health Centers. (2009, March). Primary care access: an essential building block of health care reform. Retrieved August 25, 2013, from http://www.nachc.com/client/documents/pressreleases/PrimaryCareAccessRPT.pdf

National Patient Advocate Foundation. (2012, September). Issue brief: Medical debt, medical bankruptcy and the impact on patients. The Patient's Voice. Retrieved September 5, 2013, from http://www.npaf.org/files/Medical%20Debt%20White%20Paper%20Final_0.pdf

New England Healthcare Institute (June 16, 2008). Leading health care research organizations to examine emergency department overuse. Press release. Retrieved on August 25, 2013, from http://www.nehi.net/news/press_rewlease/33/leading_health_care_research_organizations_to_examine_emergency_department_overuse

Nolte, E. & McKee, M. (2003). Measuring the health of nations: Analysis of mortality amenable to health care. British Medical Journal. 327:1129. Retrieved August 25, 2013, from http://www.bmj.com/content/327/7424/1129

Pettypiece, S. (2012, November 19). Hospital medicare cash lures doctors as costs increase. Bloomberg.com. Retrieved September 5, 2013, from http://www.bloomberg.com/news/2012-11-19/hospital-medicare-cash-lures-doctors-as-costs-increase.html

Potter, W. (2010). Deadly Spin: An insurance company insider speaks out on how corporate PR is killing health care and deceiving Americans. Bloomsbury. New York, NY

Rocky Mountain Insurance Information Association. (n.d.) Crash Costs and Statistics. RMIIA.com. Retrieved September 5, 2013, from http://www.rmiia.org/auto/traffic_safety/Cost_of_crashes.asp

Schoen, C, Lippa, J., Collins, S. & Radley, D. (2012, December). State trends in premiums and deductibles, 2003-2011: Eroding protection and rising costs underscore need for action. In Realizing Health Reform's Potential. The Commonwealth Fund, publication 1648, Vol. 31. Retrieved August 25, 2013, from http://www.commonwealthfund.org/~/media/Files/Publications/Issue%20Brief/2012/Dec/premiums/1648_Schoen_state_trends_premiums_deductibles_2003_2011_1210.pdf

Schroeder, S.A. (1979, January). The increasing use of emergency services: Why has it occurred? Is it a problem. Western Journal of Medicine 130 (1): 67-69.

Squires, D.A. (2012, May). Explaining high health care spending in the United States: An international comparison of supply, utilization, prices, and quality. The Commonwealth Fund, publication 1595, Vol. 10. Retrieved August 25, 2013 from http://www.commonwealthfund.org/Publications/Issue-Briefs/2012/May/High-Health-Care-Spending.aspx

The Physicians Foundation. (2010, October). Health reform and the decline of physician private practice: A white paper examining the effects of the patient protection and affordable care act on physician practices in the United States. Merritt Hawkins. Retrieved August 25, 2013, from http://www.physiciansfoundation.org/uploads/default/Health_Reform_and_the_Decline_of_Physcian_Private_Practice.pdf

U.S. Census Bureau (2010, September 28). Highlights: 2009. Retrieved August 25, 2013, from http://www.census.gov/hhes/www/hlthins/data/incpovhlth/2009/highlights.html

U.S. Census Bureau (2012, September 12). Highlights: 2011. Retrieved August 25, 2013, from https://www.census.gov/hihes/www/hithins/data/incpovhlth/2011/highlights.html

U.S. Department of Transporation. (2009). Traffic Safety Facts. National Highway Traffic Safety Administration National Center for Statistics and Analysis. Retrieved August 23, 2013, from http://www-nrd.nhtsa.dot.gov/Pubs/811392.pdf

Weber, E.J., et al. (2008) Are the uninsured responsible for the increase in emergency department visits in the United States. Journal of Emergency Medicine. 20 (10): 1-8.

Wikipedia.org (2013, July 26). Passenger vehicles in the United States. Retrieved August 25, 2013, from http://en.wikipedia.org/wiki/Passenger_vehicles_in_the_United_States

Woolhandler, S., Himmelstein, D., Adams, G. & Almberg, M. (2012, September 12). Despite slight drop in uninsured, last year's figure points to 48,000 preventable deaths. Physicians for a National Health Program. Retrieved August 25, 2013, from http//www.pnhp.org/news/2012/September/despite-slight-drop-in-uninsured-las-year's-figure-points-to-48000-preventable-

World Health Organization. (2011). World health statistics 2011. Global Health Observatory. Retrieved September 5, 2013, from http://www.who.int/gho/publications/world_health_statistics/2011/en/index.html

Zacks Equity Research. (2012, July 27). Health insurance stock outlook – July 2012. Retrieved September 5, 2013, from http://www.zacks.com/commentary/22522/Health-Insurance-Stock-Outlook-July-2012